Men and Menstruatio.

"A book on menstruation by a man? The clear answer, in this case, is YES. Readers, men and women alike, who can bypass doubts and the impulse to joke will find a treasure of information and wisdom in this fascinating, beautifully written account of how both sexes, together, invent the meaning of menstruation and their responses to it. The witty introduction ('Menses and Me') is worth the price of the book alone, but David Linton goes on to show how menstruation is dealt with in film, TV, ads, books, songs, and humor. 'Guys are really clueless!' one student told him. This book will clue them in. Women, too."
—Carol Tavris, Ph.D., author of *The Mismeasure of Woman* and *Anger: The Misunderstood Emotion*; coauthor of *Estrogen Matters* and *Mistakes Were Made (but not by me)*

"Many believe that menstruation is 'lady business.' Not so. Menstruation's complicated and often contradictory meanings are made through what David Linton dubs, 'the menstrual transaction.' Indeed, men have been a part of the conversation all along, but their role has been limited to that of outsiders, myth makers and antagonists who either run for the hills or weaponize their ignorance and discomfort. *We can do better.* The shifting of men (and boys) from menstrual bullies to menstrual allies requires a good hard look at the various texts that transform a bodily process into so much more. A great place to start is Linton's carefully curated tour through the sometimes painful, often funny and always illuminating menstrual discourses that leave no doubt we can and we must rewrite the rules."
—Chris Bobel, Ph.D., author of *New Blood: Third Wave Feminism and the Politics of Menstruation* and *The Managed Body: Developing Girls and Menstrual Health in the Global South*

"In a tour de force, David Linton explores the presence (and absence) of menstruation in both high and low culture. Linton's comprehensive and witty examination of men's reactions to menstruation in daily life, as well as in various forms of media, is a capstone of his thirty years of scholarly work on the topic. I can recommend this entertaining and accessible book to a broad range of readers with interests in popular culture, sex education, and gender and women's studies."
—Joan C. Chrisler, Ph.D., editor of *Women's Reproductive Health*

Men and Menstruation

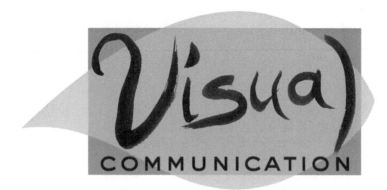

COMMUNICATION

Susan B. Barnes
General Editor

Vol. 8

The Visual Communication series
is part of the Peter Lang Media and Communication list.
Every volume is peer reviewed and meets
the highest quality standards for content and production.

PETER LANG
New York • Bern • Berlin
Brussels • Vienna • Oxford • Warsaw

David Linton

Men and Menstruation

A Social Transaction

PETER LANG
New York • Bern • Berlin
Brussels • Vienna • Oxford • Warsaw

Library of Congress Cataloging-in-Publication Control Number: 2018053965

Bibliographic information published by **Die Deutsche Nationalbibliothek**.
Die Deutsche Nationalbibliothek lists this publication in the "Deutsche
Nationalbibliografie"; detailed bibliographic data are available
on the Internet at http://dnb.d-nb.de/.

ISSN 2153-277X
ISBN 978-1-4331-5041-8 (hardcover)
ISBN 978-1-4331-6872-7 (paperback)
ISBN 978-1-4331-5042-5 (ebook pdf)
ISBN 978-1-4331-5043-2 (epub)
ISBN 978-1-4331-5044-9 (mobi)
DOI 10.3726/b12018

© 2019 Peter Lang Publishing, Inc., New York
29 Broadway, 18th floor, New York, NY 10006
www.peterlang.com

Printed in the United States of America

Contents

Acknowledgments

This book would not have been possible were it not for women. Without knowing it initially, I needed the permission and encouragement of women in order to write about a topic that is thought to be off limits to men. But once I made it clear that I had no intention to presume to speak *for* women or even *about* women but only about how women and men related to one another around the unique phenomenon of the menstrual cycle and how the interaction that I came to call "the menstrual transaction" was constructed across time and cultures and through media of communications, I was gratified to discover that women were willing to share their stories and their insights. Those sharings have been indispensable in doing the research and framing the analysis that have resulted in this book as well as many other aspects of my academic and creative endeavors.

I was first inspired to think seriously about the social construction and literary representation of menstruation by the path-breaking work of Dana Medoro which then led to my participation in a conference at the University of Liverpool titled "Menstruation: Blood, Body, Brand." This was my first exposure to others who were studying the subject and it resulted in the formation of a long-lasting friendship with another scholar, Jutta Ahlbeck, who was conducting research on menstrual education in Finland and who later hosted a conference in Turku, Finland where I had the honor of speaking. Soon I discovered the Society for Menstrual Cycle Research (SMCR), the premier professional association dedicated to examining every possible facet of the cycle. Since first attending the group's conference in 2003, members of the SMCR have become the primary source of guidance for my studies and, in fact, for the direction my career has taken.

Chief among the individuals I have to thank within the SMCR are the leaders who have invited me to speak at conferences and who have included me in the Society's endeavors, including appointing me to edit the newsletter, serve on conference planning committees, contribute to its journal and blog, and co-host one of its conferences. Those leaders include Peggy Stubbs, Chris Bobel, Ingrid Johnston-Robledo, Elizabeth Kissling, Jerrilynn Prior, Laura Werschler, Tomi-Ann Roberts, Joan Chrisler, and Evelina Sterling. The SMCR conferences are among the most stimulating events I have ever attended and I thank the many attendees and presenters who have inspired my thinking, and in particular that includes Josefin Persdotter who arranged for my stint at the University of Gothenberg in Sweden and the opportunity to engage with my host, Professor Cathrin Wasshede, and the other Swedish scholars there.

My training in the Media Ecology Department at New York University accomplished what a good education is supposed to do: it taught me how to think more clearly and provided a set of lenses through which to view every aspect of communications and media experiences, even though I wasn't studying menstruation at the time. For this I owe a debt of gratitude to Neil Postman and Christine Nystrom, my mentors and role models, as well as to the many classmates who contributed to my growth.

I have had the privilege of working for nearly 30 years at Marymount Manhattan College, a school where curiosity was respected and rewarded. The rewards included research support, opportunities to teach course on this unusual topic, students who challenged my ideas and contributed to my understanding, colleagues who validated my interests and suggested new ways to look at the subject. Three Academic Deans—Dawn Weber, Paula Mayhew, and Ann Jablon—supported my teaching and scholarship. Special thanks are offered to present and former members of the Communication Arts Department; Katie LeBesco, Laura Tropp, Jenny Dixon, Giovanna Chessler, Peter Schaefer, Alistir Sanderson, and especially MJ Robinson, a long-time office mate and bulwark against folly and pretension.

Sadly, space and the limits of memory to not allow the identification of the long list of students who have influenced my thinking with their insights and willingness to share personal stories that shed light on the subject we studied together. In some cases I have had the opportunity to extend the teacher-student relationship beyond graduation into ongoing friendships and further efforts to better understanding the endlessly fascinating topic of the social construction of menstruation. We have become colleagues and co-learners. Among those wonderful

ACKNOWLEDGMENTS | IX

ex-students are Kelly Renn, Sarah Peterson, Robyn Percyz, Emily Swann, Carly Schneider, and Julia Matarazzo. Saniya Ghanoui has transitioned from student to co-author, co-presenter, co-planner and good friend.

Thanks for their patience and support is due to Susan Barnes, Series Editor, and Kathryn Harrison and Erika Hendrix, Acquisitions Editors, at Peter Lang Publishing. They make an author feel one is in good hands.

Finally, this book could not have been conceived of, let alone written, without the presence of Simi Linton in my life. She has deeply enriched my understanding of what it means to be a woman and, by sharing her life with me and inviting me to share my life with her, has broadened my understanding of myself as a man as well as my understanding of being human.

Introduction

Menses and Me

This book is about men and menstruation, about how men and women relate to each other around the presence of the period. (Note: Though some transgender individuals who have transitioned from female to male continue to menstruate, for purposes of social and cultural analysis, the term "women" will be used to refer to people who have, have had, or will have menstrual cycles.) Drawing upon personal experience, interviews, and an examination of how the period is presented in film, TV, advertising, literature, song lyrics, and humor, the following pages reveal that the meaning of menstruation is something that men and women invent together through an endless series of "menstrual transactions."

My own earliest memory of anything menstrual occurred when I was about ten years old. It was just before my father's birthday; I'd gotten him a bulky sweater but had nothing to wrap it in. One day as I was leaving the bathroom I noticed a pale blue and white box on the top of the trash basket; I picked it up, carrying it into the dining room as my mother came by. "What are you going to do with that?" she asked.

"I'm going to use it to wrap Dad's sweater in. It's just the right size."

"No, you can't use that," she said.

"Why not? I don't have anything else."

"You can't use that," she insisted. "Find something else."

Now my antennae were quivering. Something was going on here. "Why not? What is this?"

We parried back and forth a few more times, and then she said some magic words, an incantation that brought the conversation to a halt, "It's something I use."

There was power and mystery in her words and the way she said them. I sensed that the pale blue box with the words *feminine napkins* on it had to do with being a woman, something that I was not allowed to know, not just because I was a kid but because there were things about all women that all men, whether boys or grown men, were forbidden to know. I returned the box to the trash basket and dropped the subject. As I recall that moment, I wish I'd wrapped Dad's sweater in the box without Mom knowing, that I'd wrapped it with "Happy Birthday!" tissue. If only I could have seen Dad's reaction upon encountering the box. Would he have been amused? Would he or Mom have been embarrassed? Would they have covered the awkwardness with laughter or blushes? To my recollection, the subject never again came up and I remember nothing more about the presence of the period in my home.

Years later the period took on new meaning and led to the writing of this book. My main inspiration came from Prince Charles, heir to the Throne of England (described in detail in Chapter 3). A brief news item in 1993 reported (falsely, it turned out) that a secretly taped phone conversation between Charles and his lover (now wife) Camilla included a fantasy in which he longed to be reincarnated as a tampon so he could reside within her. When I mentioned the story to my wife, she said, "See? That's the difference between men and women. Men think there's something erotic about inserting a tampon. Women never think that way. It's like the way men imagine there's something erotic about a gynecological exam. Women don't think that having a pelvic exam is sexy."

The conversation got me thinking about the different ways that women and men view the period, and I wondered what Alfred Kinsey, the father of modern sex research, had discovered. To my surprise, upon looking up "menstruation" in both Kinsey volumes, *Sexual Behavior in the Human Male* (1948) and *Sexual Behavior in the Human Female* (1953), I discovered that Kinsey virtually skipped the topic completely.

In the earliest volume on male sexual behavior he gave ample attention (with many charts and graphs) to correlations between variables such as age, education level, religious background, etc. and frequency of sexual activity including masturbation, morning erections, intercourse and other related means of sexual satisfaction and engagement. However, there is not a single mention of how or if male sexual activity is related to the menstrual status of their partners. Despite the fact that it is well known that many religious and cultural traditions place restrictions on intercourse with a menstruating woman, Kinsey made no mention of how such circumstances affected frequency, let alone the possible impact on the variations in activity employed to accommodate the aesthetic reactions individuals might have to genital contact with menstrual blood or the practical matter of dealing with the stains that are likely to result.

Even in reporting on women's sexual behavior five years later Kinsey gave no indication that having a period had any effect on women's intercourse practices. Once again, the volume has a plethora of charts and graphs chronicling variables such as age at first sexual experience and first period, education level, age at the onset of menopause, etc. In a section where one might have expected a discussion of how menstruation sometimes curtails sexual activity—a mention of "restraining factors," those conditions that contribute to curtailing sexual activity—there is mention of religion and fear of pregnancy but not of having one's period. However, there are some other menstrual related data, such as the fact that menopause may account for an increase in sexual activity due to being "relieved of the possibility of becoming pregnant" (p. 735). And there is a by now antiquated use of the term "female castration" to refer to women who have had their ovaries surgically removed and no longer menstruate. Kinsey reported that for such women there is "no modification of sexual responsiveness or capacity for orgasm" (p. 734).

Given the thoroughness of the Kinsey research team's examination of a vast array of behaviors, the absence of menstrual investigations was striking. One of the purposes of this book is to fill the gaps that Kinsey left unexplored.

What was it about menstruation and sex—or about Kinsey—that made him leave out anything having to do with how couples negotiated their sexual practices around the period? Or was it that he did the research but decided to omit it from the published volume, perhaps in fear of provoking even more controversy than the publications were already guaranteed to engender? The latter possibility was eliminated during the first of several visits I made to the Kinsey Institute at the University of Indiana. I asked the archivist in charge of Kinsey's case study files about the omission of details about menstrual relations. He stared at me for a moment in surprise before acknowledging that he'd never noticed its absence. The next day, having reviewed the archives, he confirmed my observation and confessed that no one had ever pointed this out before. My smug pleasure at having found a lapse in Kinsey's research soon gave way to a deeper curiosity as to why he missed it and, more important, what was actually going on in the menstrual lives of women and men anyway?

However, before trying to fathom the private details of other people's menstrual lives and how their views and values were formed, I decided that I should first try to reconstruct my own experiences, what I've come to call "menstrual history." How did I learn about the period, what did I know about my mother's cycle, how had my own sex life been affected by the menstrual cycles of women I had been involved with? Other than the story about my mother and the mysterious box, I was surprised to discover how sketchy my memories were. Eventually I recalled several encounters that shaped my values and ways of dealing with the period's presence in my life.

Following my mother's secretive behavior, my next menstrual encounter occurred some years later at the age of 16. My girlfriend Terri and I had done some mutual groping though I wasn't at all clear about what was actually "down there." One day she informed me on the phone that we couldn't "do anything" that afternoon because of "the 13th letter." She responded to my confusion by spelling out "m-e-n-s-t-r-u-a-t-i-o-n," a word she wouldn't say out loud. Being a bookish kid, I looked up the word but could make no sense of the definition so I said it aloud the next time I saw her. Terri quickly put her hand over my mouth and looked around furtively, though we were sitting alone on the railroad tracks behind her house. And when I tried to touch her, she reminded me, "No, it's the 13th letter. We have to wait till next week." Shortly afterwards Terri broke up with me (an older boy with a car had more appeal) so my education was cut short for the time being.

It wasn't until my junior year in college that another menstrual concern arose. My girlfriend and I had our first intercourse, unprotected and rushed, one night in my apartment while my roommates were away. I was thrilled that we'd moved beyond our long months of furtive petting and the next day set about buying condoms as I looked ahead to a new stage in our sex life.

Two weeks later when I met her at the dorm, she said, "I'm late." I have since come to understand that these are among the two most frightening words in the English language, but at the time my oblivion was so complete I simply replied, "That's OK, I just got here myself."

"No," she said, "I mean, I'm LATE. I didn't get my period."

In retrospect I think I could have been an apt argument for why sex education should be a school requirement. I hadn't given a single thought to the possibility that the sudden emission I'd had two weeks earlier could have any consequences. She told me she had an appointment with a doctor in two days and would tell me the outcome afterwards. We didn't discuss the situation any further.

If "I'm late" are words that can make the heart race in fear, then there are three others that can elicit elation. Two days later I heard those words as my girlfriend raced across Oak Grove in the center of the campus to announce, "I got it!" All of our contraceptive practices for the next twelve years (condoms, foams, diaphragms, pills, and eventually my vasectomy) were so thorough that I never again heard that scary sentence.

By the time I was in my early 30s I thought I understood how the period worked and what it meant to women. But that was before *Star Wars* came out.

I loved that movie. I was knocked out by the establishing shot of Luke Skywalker's home planet on which we see, off in the distance, Luke's hovercraft zooming across a barren landscape of literally unearthly colors and terrain. But the most striking element in that scene was the fact that there appeared to be two moons in the sky. As I recall it, one was a full, perfect circle of glowing yellow in a dark sky, the other only partially visible, in a different lunar phase. I was thrilled to think of how different a sky would look with two or more moons, and our own solitary orb suddenly seemed plain and dull by comparison.

For weeks I regaled friends with my wonder over this stimulating prospect. Then one day I described the scene to a woman who promptly replied, "Wow, can you imagine what periods would be like on that planet!" This idea startled me even more than the thought of more complex tidal charts, bright nights, plant growth, nocturnal animal behavior or navigational variations. It was another moment when I realized that women experienced the world differently than I did and that one of the influences that shaped perspectives was menstruation. My friend was as much a resident of another planet as was Luke Skywalker. Her "otherness" was as vivid and as memorable as that of the movie's Wookies and Jedi Knights.

Looking back on that conversation, I now understand more clearly what I merely suspected then. The way the presence of the period functions in our social lives is both unique and general. Virtually all people—men and women alike—have menstrual memories; both parties—as individuals and as classes—share in shaping the meanings of the differences between the individuals and the groups they belong to. The same is true of race, gender, class, and every other division we use to sort people, but no matter which group we're assigned to, we still participate somehow in the ones outside.

At the same time as my *Star Wars* moment, my own menstrual consciousness continued to evolve, as I was single in those years. My sexual relationships were mostly unaffected by whether or not a partner was menstruating, though sometimes early in a relationship women were reluctant to engage in menstrual sex until some emotional intimacy had been established. Sometimes I found that women would tentatively mention the period's presence to see if that was OK with me and to make sure we adequately managed sheet protection and clean up. I do recall one amusing miscommunication. I was seeing a woman who lived some distance away; she'd arranged to come visit for a weekend, and I phoned a few days in advance to work out her travel plans. She sounded a little cool during the conversation, and finally said, "I'm not sure I should come. I have my friend this week." I misread her completely and said, "Oh, that's all right. Bring her along."

My date's past experience with men's negative views and her own reservations made her misread me as well, "Are you sure? You don't mind?"

"No, of course not." I answered. "It'll be fun. I'm sure we'll have a good time."

She sounded pleased and perked up as we made arrangements to meet at the train station. When she arrived alone, I asked, with some disappointment, "Where's your friend? Did she decide not to come?"

"What friend?"

"You said you were bringing your friend with you."

"Huh? ..." Suddenly, she got it. "No, I meant, you know *my friend*." She surrounded the words with fingered air quotes.

Now, finally, I got it too. We both laughed and I told her that her friend was welcome in any form and we went on to have a great weekend together with plenty of joking references to our mutual confusion.

Since then, I've become an active observer of the dynamics surrounding the period, constantly alert for its subtle presence in our midst, gathering stories that others have to tell of their own confusions, accidents, pleasures, and discoveries. It's surprising how willing people are to talk about menstruation once they've been given an invitation to do so by a curious listener. For example, consider this story about the best menstrual joke I've ever heard, memorable in part because of the circumstances in which I heard it and the story surrounding it.

One evening at dinner with a small group of friends, including a couple in their mid-20s, the subject of my research came up. I explained that I was interested in how men and women dealt with the period in their lives, and the young woman told me a story about a friend of hers, a woman of her age, who'd recently completed her MBA and was interviewing for jobs with various corporations. The friend was a petite blond with a demure manner and conservative appearance. She went through a rigorous series of interviews at a major financial firm known for its hard-charging, frat boy corporate culture. When she reached the final round, she found herself in a large office with the top executive of the division, a forbidding, middle-aged man, who said, "You're obviously well qualified and can probably do the job. But I'd like to get some idea of what you're like personally. How about telling me a joke." Without a moment's hesitation, the candidate responded with the following:

It was the night of the Palace Ball and Cinderella desperately wanted to attend. Her Fairy Godmother had provided her with a gown and beautiful dancing slippers, but Cinderella told her that she had one additional problem, "I'm on my period and I have a very heavy flow. I don't have anything that can handle it." Her

Fairy Godmother replied, "Don't worry. I'll give you a magic tampon, the most absorbent tampon ever created, but there is one condition. You must return home by midnight or it will turn into a pumpkin."

Cinderella took the magic tampon and went off to the ball. As midnight approached, the Fairy Godmother and stepsisters waited anxiously for Cinderella's return. Midnight passed, and then one, two, and three o'clock. Finally, at dawn, Cinderella arrived home in a royal carriage smiling blissfully and collapsed into a chair. Everyone gathered around, eager to hear about her adventures and concerned for her wellbeing. "I had a wonderful time!" she exclaimed. "I met a handsome prince, and we danced and partied all night." Her Fairy Godmother interrupted to ask, "What was his name?" Cinderella smiled and replied, "Peter, Peter Pumpkin Eater."

Now, as jokes go, this may or may not be a great one. I find it funny both for its set up (a magic tampon) and its pay off on Peter the Pumpkin Eater (naturally, she would meet other fairy tale characters at a fairy tale ball). But the circumstances of its telling—both in the business office and the restaurant where I heard it retold—are culturally revealing. The unassuming, conservative-appearing job applicant hitting a prospective male boss with an oral sex menstrual joke was her way of letting him know that she was tough and daring, a risk taker who was not shy and wasn't afraid to assert her right to be a woman—and a tough one at that. And she got the job.

The second part of the transaction was the telling of the story to me by the young woman I'd just met. She too, like her friend, was at ease with menstruation and used the story to let me know so. In fact, I believe that she may have even been taking the initiative to put me at ease with her.

One way of summarizing the questions that these personal stories suggest is to ask, "What's with the men in menstruation?" By now questions about my own menstrual history have become more general. Now I want to know what kinds of menstrual experience and stories do men have in common? One way of answering that question is to find out how male encounters with the period have been treated in novels, films, poems, and TV shows.

In pursuit of an answer to that question I've read dozens of stories that include menstrual transactions and have studied such scenes in numerous movies and TV shows. Though stories with menstrual details are uncommon, when looked at as a group they are fascinating. Some of the chapters in this book are devoted to those examples. I've also interviewed dozens of men and women about their menstrual histories and devote separate chapters to their stories as well. But as a preview, let me mention the two themes that run through the tales I've been told.

For women, the common theme has to do with embarrassment: every woman I've spoken with has a story to tell about her own or a friend's "accident," a stained skirt, a mark on a chair, an insensitive male teacher who denied permission to go to the girls' room at a crucial time. Sometimes the stories include details of the strategies invented to handle a "leak," or how young girls make up secret menstrual language, or check out each other's rear ends to insure safety. The phrase "I've got your back" is not just appropriate to street gangs or soldiers looking out for one another.

The common theme for men has to do with a mysterious incident, much like my story about the feminine napkin box—an encounter that left them asking, "What's going on here? What am I not supposed to know?" Two examples: a researcher asked pre-adolescent boys what they knew about the period. The most memorable reply was from the boy who responded, "We don't know what it is but we know we're supposed to be nice to girls when they have it." The other example concerns a male student of mine who described coming home from high school one day and discovering his 12-year-old sister in her room crying in pain and being comforted by her mother. He went to his father and asked, "Is Elizabeth going to die?" The father's vague answer, "No, this is just something that happens to women sometimes," relieved him of his fear but left him confused about why she was in misery.

Once I'd conducted a good deal of research, examined hundreds of magazine and TV ads and given many talks at conferences, I decided to offer a course for college students so I could better organize and share what I'd learned and benefit from the insights that students would bring to the conversation. I created a course called "The Social Construction and Images of Menstruation" to be offered as an elective for upper level students at the liberal arts college where I teach. I had no idea if students would enroll, but to my delight it filled quickly with 19 women and two men. It quickly became a staple of the curriculum.

The first semester I approached the course nervously; making a group of undergraduates comfortable with a senior male faculty member talking about the menstrual cycle was a new challenge. One particular student turned out to be the most valuable resource I had. Yvonne was what we sometimes call a "returning woman" student, a woman in her middle years who'd raised a family, relocated from Detroit to New York, and set out to complete a college degree long ago begun and abandoned. She sat in the front row and was not the least bit shy about explaining to the 20-year-olds the differences in the ways her generations had been educated (or not!) about their cycles and the real-life effects of menopause, hysterectomy and other personal details that I could only discuss in the most abstract, impersonal, and textbook-based fashion.

Yvonne's most memorable comment occurred the day we were discussing the historical, religious, and psychological bases for the taboos against having sex during the period. One young woman asked, "I don't get it. Don't men always want to have sex?"

Yvonne turned slowly to face the class, smiled wisely, and responded, "Just wait."

I've now taught the course more than twenty times. It's been the most rewarding experience in all my years of teaching. Previously I'd created courses and published articles on topics as diverse as educational media, the Luddite movement, Shakespeare, the Virgin Mary, film studies, and media history. But now my family refers to that body of work as part of my "pre-menstrual period." In "the period class" (as students call it) every day brings a new insight or an illuminating story as students learn to link seemingly trivial observations to larger, historically or sociologically significant themes. Each session typically begins with someone saying, "Wait till you hear this one!"

Consider the following examples. "Guys are really clueless!" a young woman exclaimed one day. "My roommate had the weirdest date this weekend. She was at a restaurant with a new guy and was trying to find something in her bag and she dumped a bunch of stuff out on the table, including an eyelash curler. The guy got all excited and said, 'What are you doing?! You can't have that thing out here. Put that away!' She asked him what he was talking about and he pointed to the curler. 'Put that away. That's disgusting!' She finally got him to tell her what was the matter. He thought it was some kind of tampon extractor!"

Of course, everyone in the class was both amused and appalled at the fellow's dismay. The story led to an excellent conversation about male ignorance about women's business, including both make-up and menstrual technology. Then we turned to consideration of how in the world he made up or learned such a strange idea; since the woman didn't date the guy again (his expression of disgust repelled her), we couldn't ask her to go back and ask him, so we came up with two hypotheses. The first was that since he may have known that some sort of insertion device or applicator was commonly used to place the tampon within the vagina, then it must require some sort of extractor to take it out. The second idea was that perhaps he'd seen some film or pictures having to do with gynecological exams that included images of a speculum. The devices do have a vague resemblance to each other and he may have leapt to that conclusion. The larger point was how many ways men and women are unaware of the details of one another's lives and how and why such a condition reinforces expectations and behaviors.

Another story concerns a celebrity, and even comes with a sequel. "I work as an usher at a Broadway theater," the student began. "Last Wednesday I was working the matinee and after everyone was seated after intermission I went down to the women's room to change my tampon. As I walked in with my tampon in my hand, Catherine Zeta Jones was sitting at the make-up table. She looked up and said, 'Yeah, me too. Ain't it a bother?' We traded a few complaints about cramps and bloating and then went into adjacent cubicles. And then, I could hear Catherine Zeta Jones tearing open her tampon wrapper!!"

We got past this charming story of an encounter with a menstruating star and dug into its meaning, that women's menstrual bonding transcends boundaries of class, status, celebrity, wealth and just about any other barrier we could think of. Then I asked, "What do men have like this?"

After a long pause someone reluctantly asked, "Sports?" Class members generally agreed that for men sport conversation worked in very similar ways, so I pushed the association a bit further to discuss a piece of graffiti once seen in a women's bathroom: "Sports and war are menstrual envy." At first the idea was met with skepticism but it became the opportunity to explore the counter-point to Freud's notion of penis envy, variously called menstrual envy or womb envy. Although no one became thoroughly convinced, it gave us yet another opportunity to look into the nuances of menstrual culture.

The sequel to the story happened five weeks later during the first session following the Thanksgiving break. "So I went home for the holiday," the student began, "and I told my mom and dad separately about meeting Catherine Zeta Jones, but I left out the menstrual details when I spoke with my dad. The next day at a large family dinner my dad said, 'Tell everyone about who you met at the theater!' My mother looked at me and rolled her eyes and I thought, you know, I'm taking this class and I'm learning that there's nothing shameful about the period, so I decided to tell the full story. When I got to the point about taking my tampon to the women's room, a weird thing happened. All the women at the table leaned forward and all the men leaned back. And then my Dad said, 'I don't need to hear this,' and left the table."

Not only was this a sequel to the celebrity story, it was a natural follow up on research the students had recently completed that required them to conduct a set of interviews with other individuals about their menstrual histories. The assignment didn't ask them to find out about "flow" or biological details of the period but about how men and women relate to each other around the period.

The interview assignment has turned out to be the most valuable one in the course. Students approach it with a mix of anxiety and enthusiasm. I save it until the last month so that by then their own comfort level has become high enough for them to feel that they can handle the awkwardness it might entail. I also tell them that if they feel uncomfortable we'll come up with an alternative assignment. So far, no one has taken that option.

The day the assignment is due is especially exciting as everyone arrives with discoveries and insights. Some are funny, others are shocking, some are sad. Everyone seems to feel proud (and sometimes a bit smug) at having arrived at a level of mature comfort greater than that with which they began the course. Many moments stand out in my memory. For instance, one particularly strong, assertive young woman was troubled at a personal discovery. "I had planned on interviewing my mother for the assignment and was looking forward to it for a month. But then every time I began to raise the subject, I couldn't do it. I realized that we'd never talked about my period and I couldn't bring myself to ask her about hers. I always thought my Mom and I had a very open relationship, but now I realize it's a lot more complicated or one way."

Some students interview the whole family—father, mother, siblings and grandparents. They discover generational differences in education, attitude, knowledge and views about products, such as the older generation's life-long resistance to using tampons.

The course concludes with the usual term paper requirement. Perhaps a good way to relate just how rich the material is would be to list the titles of some of their papers:

- Menstrual Synchronicity: Who's the Lead Bleeder?
- Menstrual Practices in Ethiopia (or, any other place)
- The Evolution of Menstrual Product Advertising
- The Ballerina and Amenorrhea
- Menstruation Management in Prisons
- Who's Fit for the Flow?—Menstruation and Sterilization
- The Horror of Menstruation: Menses in Horror Movies
- What's in Your Tampon? (an analysis of chemical content)
- Turning Blood Green: Environmentally Friendly Menstrual Products
- An Analysis of Menstrual Symbolism in Four Versions of *Carrie*
- Cross-Cultural Menstrual Superstitions and Taboos
- Menstrual Sex: Exploring the Taboo

There is one more way that "The Period Class" is different from any other that I've taught. Well after the course is over and students have graduated, many stay in touch by sending me emails of occasional "sightings," as we've come to call them: photos of tampon Halloween costumes, a story of shopping for tampons in Egypt, playing the menstrual card to beat a traffic ticket. Throughout my career there have always been students I've stayed in touch with, but this seems different. These students take a special pride in their enhanced observational skills and feel special, almost as though they belong to a secret society that sets them apart from others with less menstrual savvy.

The Prince Charles story that I began with, and the ongoing discoveries since, have led me not only to reflections on my own menstrual history, but I've also come to believe that the way individual men and women view the period encapsulates some core values about the way they see essential qualities of male and female character. I've come to believe that though the menstrual cycle is a biological phenomenon that has existed since our earliest humanoid development (despite changes wrought by differences in nutrition and child bearing), its meaning has been constructed and revised in an infinite variety of ways to suit the social, religious, economic, or aesthetic needs of the people of any given culture. I've come to believe that in contemporary American society menstrual attitudes are determined largely by economic imperatives, as now we see a competition between the makers of pads and tampons, the drug industries that produce menstrual suppression products, and new arrivals on the scene: menstrual cups, reusable pads, and specially designed "period panties," not to mention a fervent activism devoted to "outing" the period. And I've come to believe that we are presently undergoing an historic series of changes in the menstrual ecology that are driven by both social circumstances and pharmaceutical advances, and that these changes have consequences of their own, many of which are unanticipated and unpredictable.

For nearly twenty years, as a teacher, as a writer, and simply as a man who has developed an abiding fascination with the apparently infinite variety of ways that societies and individuals have imposed layers of meaning upon a fundamental biological "fact of live," I have been striving to better understand "the period." Currently I serve on the Board of the Society for Menstrual Cycle Research and co-edit its newsletter, *The Periodical*. I have hosted its biennial conference, serve on the editorial board of its journal, *Women's Reproductive Health*, and have written nearly one hundred posts for its blog, *Menstruation Matters* as well as articles in scholarly journals. Some of the following material has been previously published in other venues over the course of my studies.

As an additional means of exploring and better expressing my understanding of the menstrual transaction I have written a series of poems on the topic that I have titled *The Menstrual Odyssey*. The collection imagines a span of time, beginning with a cave man's earliest encounter with menstrual blood, and concluding with poetic snap shots of how contemporary men respond to it. It also depicts the range of reactions that males might have from pre-pubescent menstrual encounters through adolescence and adulthood. I have performed many of these works at venues such as the London Poetry Society Café, The Bowery Poetry Club, The Neuyorican Café, and many other settings both in the U.S. and abroad.

To put it simply, the meaning of menstruation has been and continues to be the most intriguing, intellectually engaging, and personally rewarding subject I have ever encountered.

Finally, I think it is important to mention that this book makes no claim to being an exhaustive study of the topic. And I make no claim to speak for women's experiences with menstruation. There is a wealth of research, scholarship, criticism, personal reflection, film, art, and other material created by women that articulates the perception of those who actually experience a menstrual cycle. Furthermore, the remarkable activism that women have engaged in to challenge the stereotypes and ignorance surrounding menstruation deserves mention and praise: legislative initiatives to require safe manufacturing practices and testing of menstrual products; drives to eliminate sales taxes on pads and tampons; campaigns to require the provision of free products in schools shelters, and prisons; educational initiatives to offer better understanding of the biology of menstruation; rallies to defy gender stereotype These and so many more endeavors have been created and carried out by women dedicated to eliminating the ways that one aspect of women's biology, their menstrual cycle, have been used to deny them the rightful participation in every aspect of life on both the social and personal level.

References

Kinsey, A., Pomeroy, W., & Martin, C. (1948). *Sexual behavior in the human male*. Philadelphia, PA: W.B. Saunders.
Kinsey, A., Pomeroy, W., Martin, C., & Gebhard, P. (1953). *Sexual behavior in the human female*. Philadelphia, PA: W.B. Saunders.

PART I

Men and the Menstrual Landscape

At first glance it might seem that men would have little to do with deciding how to view the menstrual cycle, how to manage its regular occurrence, how women and men should behave in its presence. But in societies where men decide what virtually everything means, from seemingly trivial matters such as hair styles and clothing choices to one's notions of god and eternity, and even how and when to have sexual intercourse, then it is unavoidable that men would play a part in deciding how to manage the monthly appearance of menstrual fluid that women experience.

The first three chapters of this book delve into wide ranging aspects of male encounters with menstruation. The first chapter introduces the concept of "the menstrual transaction," how men and women jointly participate in shaping their relationships in a menstrual context. The second chapter offers a perspective on how the ancient religious traditions that lie at the heart of Islam, Judaism, and Christianity defined menstruation and describes the three Biblical incidents involving menstruating women that shaped the Christian faith. The third chapter is a case study of one man's unfortunate encounter with the menstrual rules of order and how it affected his public image, the sad saga of Charles, Prince of Wales.

CHAPTER ONE

The Menstrual Transaction

"If you be not mad, begone; if you have reason, be brief. 'Tis not that time of moon with me to make one in so skipping a dialogue."

Olivia to Viola/Cesario
Twelfth Night—Act I, Scene 5
William Shakespeare

The encounter cited above suggests that 16th-century Elizabethans had their own issues around occasional menstrual discomfort and that Shakespeare knew he could get a laugh out of alluding to the matter. The subject is given an additional spin by the fact that Olivia's brazen mention of her menstrual cycle to a person she believed to be a young man named Cesario (though actually a woman in disguise named Viola, one of Shakespeare's many forays into gender bending flirtations; today the play stands as a disquisition on the politics of passing, identity and gender fluidity) is used as a means of demonstrating her hauteur as well as her superior social status. The playwright's full intention behind this piece of dialogue cannot be known, but the idea that Elizabethan women might have had periods that impacted their moods is clear, and the notion must have been common enough for its mention to be acceptable in a theatrical production, though it might have raised some hackles. This brief jape (to stay with Elizabethan style for a moment) encapsulates the impact that menstrually provoked mood changes are thought to have on the ways people, particularly men and women, relate to one another. While Shakespeare's audience may not yet have had the diagnostic terminology such as "premenstrual syndrome," they seemed familiar with the experience. Meanwhile, men have continued to bandy about their notions of the meaning of menstruation in revealing ways, right down to the realm of political discourse.

As in so many aspects of American social, political, and economic life, Donald Trump had an impact on what we might call "the menstrual ecology." His widely reported, seemingly off-hand remark criticizing TV news personality Megyn Kelly's treatment of him during one of the televised debates, "You could see there was blood coming out of her eyes, blood coming out of her—wherever" (Rucker, 2015), expressed male anxiety about the imagined power and perceived nastiness of women who are thought to be menstruating. But it also served to open such feelings to more public scrutiny. However, Donald Trump is hardly the first political leader to publicly air opinions about the presumed effects of menstruation. One of his predecessors in this realm was another head of state, Col. Mummar el-Qaddafi.

Over the course of his 42-year reign over Libya Qaddafi produced a three-part treatise titled *The Green Book* that laid out his political/social/economic theories regarding the ways society should be organized. It appears to have been somewhat modeled after Chairman Mao's *Little Red Book*. He called his conception "the Third International Theory." It is an often-rambling discourse on a wide range of topics, including the nature of men and women, education, politics and the Libyan constitution. He included in his pronouncements a lengthy treatise on proper gender roles, including mention of the part menstruation plays in human arrangements. To a critical reader his writings seem particularly bombastic and self-evident, as in the following excerpt:

> Women are females and men are males. According to gynecologists, women menstruate every month or so, while men, being male, do not menstruate or suffer during the monthly period. A woman, being a female, is naturally subject to monthly bleeding. When a woman does not menstruate, she is pregnant. If she is pregnant, she becomes, due to pregnancy, less active for about a year, which means that all her natural activities are seriously reduced until she delivers her baby. (Qaddafi, n.d.)

The point of this little biology lesson is to justify the sharp role requirements and separations of duties that Qaddafi spells out elsewhere in the document. But at least he does not attack women for their biology; rather, he is emphatic in insisting upon women's right to own property, seek divorce and in other ways claim full social and political equality. Back in the U.S. we might note a remark by another political commentator whose opinion was more in keeping with Donald Trump's.

May 27, 2009, G. Gordon Liddy, a conservative radio talk show host, convicted Watergate burglar, and Ronald Reagan campaign aide, responded to President Barak Obama's nomination of Sonia Sotomayor to fill a Supreme Court vacancy by stating, on the air, "Let's hope that the key conferences aren't when she's menstruating or something, or just before she's going to menstruate. That would really be bad. Lord knows what we would get then" (Frick, 2009).

Much ink has been spilled (and blood let) over the nature of gender differences. A strong case can be made for the idea that misogyny in its many forms (clitorectomy, foot binding, rape, and other violent acts as well as condescension, targeted sarcasm, and the other innumerable occasions of sexist acts, words and thoughts) is a reflection of male insecurity, that male bullying constitutes attempts to compensate for deep seated doubts as to one's own power or worthiness, whether it be on a personal or societal level. If, as I suspect, misogyny has its roots in fear of "otherness," and one of the two distinguishing marks of the otherness of women is the menstrual cycle (the other being child bearing), then menses predictably must be processed by men in terms of what its characteristics reveal about those without it. Another aspect of the male posture is use of menstruation as a way to dismiss a woman's argument, opinion, feelings or behavior by crediting it (or blaming it!) on her cycle, even when she is not in the pre-menstrual phase sometimes associated with mood changes or discomfort.

Menstrual insults and prejudice have a long history. Alvy Singer, Woody Allen's character in *Annie Hall*, was neither the first nor the last man to dismissively ask a woman, "What's the matter, are you on your period?" William Shakespeare depicted similar menstrual malice in *Romeo and Juliet* when Juliet's father berates his daughter for her recalcitrant response to her parents' insistence that she marry Paris:

But fettle your fine joints 'gainst Thursday next
To go with Paris to Saint Peter's Church,
Or I will drag thee on a hurdle thither.
Out, you green sickness, carrion!
Out, you baggage? You tallow face!" (Act III, Scene 5)

The term "green sickness" was an Elizabethan colloquial expression for a young girl who had a delayed menarche, and Lord Capulet attributes her defiance to a case of "female trouble," in this case the notion that Juliet had not "grown up" enough to have a period and act like a "real" woman rather than a spoiled child (Evans & Read, 2017, p. 128). From ancient times men have speculated about the mysteries of the menstrual cycle and the womb, attempting to make sense of biological functions that were so different from their own. Women's bodies were conceived as inferior deviations from male bodies. According to Evans and Read (2017), "it was assumed that they were looser and more prone to leaking than the firmer, drier male body. Medical norms also presumed that women led more sedate lives than men, so they didn't use up all their blood in the way that men did, necessitating menstruation" (p. x). The ancient Roman historian Pliny went so far as to claim that,

> menstrual blood had many startling properties, such as the ability to make a dog mad should he taste it, kill whole fields of crops, or to drive bees from their hives. It could also blunt knives, make iron go rusty, dull a mirror, and had the power to make the unwitting suitor fall in love if some of the woman's powdered blood was slipped into his drink. (p. 15)

Apparently, belief in the aphrodisiac power of menses was long lasting, as Carlo Levi makes mention of it in his tale of life in rural Southern Italy in the early 1940s (1947, p. 14).

The list of menstrual powers and unfortunate outcomes has changed over time having also included causing breast cancer and smallpox in children. Even miscarriages, birth abnormalities, and molar pregnancies, were attributed ("blamed" may be a more apt word) on the possibility that a woman engaged in intercourse while she was menstruating as such acts could result in creating a "moon calf" or even a monster. The lengths to which men have gone in order to come to grips with and to regulate the strange, foreign, frightening, and awesome capacity that women possess have been boundless.

At first consideration one might think that since men don't menstruate themselves, they would have nothing to do with the meaning and management of menstruation, but the truth has turned out just the opposite. It requires an act of sustained discipline to ignore and to stay ignorant of something as fascinating as the menstrual cycle. It takes prolonged conditioning to train men to turn off their curiosity and desire to understand nature's mysteries. For as long as human culture has existed, menstruation's mysterious "otherness" has been for men a constant source of curiosity and creative myth making across time and all human societies. Consider the plight of the cave dwellers.

For men in pre-historic times, the bleeding body of another man likely meant that he had been attacked by an animal or competing male or had taken a bad fall or had some sickening condition. In each case, blood flow was a sign of mortality: bleeding often preceded death, just as it did in the case of the animals men slew in their hunting forays (Shlain, 1993, p. 63). It must have been both terrifying and awesome—terrifying because blood flow signified death; awesome because it had no connection to injury and in a few days disappeared only to appear again from time to time. Men are still in awe, and sometimes in fear, of this occurrence, as expressed in an old joke, "Don't trust anything that can bleed for seven days and not die."

To make matters even more confusing, unlike the situation with virtually every other biological processes, there are virtually no models within the rest of the animal world from which humans can learn about this unique human characteristic as very few other species experience menstruation (Schlain, 2003, p. 17). Furthermore, unlike modern women living in industrialized societies who commonly have as many as 400 periods during their reproductive lives, it is highly likely that many pre-historic forebears had far fewer due to frequent pregnancy, extended nursing (lactation suppresses ovulation), and nutritional shortcomings (Shlain, p. 30).

Various explanations have been offered for these reactions in men, but it all comes down to the fact that, as Marie Mulvey-Roberts (2003) puts it, "menstruation generates mythologies partly because it is not understood." The desire to understand is the source of myth, lore, religion, magic, superstition, and scientific hypotheses. Since, with rare exceptions, women were the ones getting periods, for them it became "normal." In fact, Shlain (1993) postulated that the regularity of the menstrual cycle and its similarity to lunar cycles led women to be the discoverers or inventors of the very concept of "time," as they arrived at the insight that the recurrence of their cycle could be charted and predicted in tandem with the moon's phases (pp. 165–185).

Meanwhile, men have imbued it with multiple "meanings," a task that has led to an amazing variety of beliefs and social practices. Over the years men invented codes of conduct for women to abide by that turned the seemingly miraculous gift, into a social deficit, a curse that had the devilish power to spoil food, blight crops, and render unfit for social intercourse (let alone the sexual variety!) any woman so beset with the contamination. Clearly, the vast majority of menstrual beliefs and practices were created by men: how else can we explain how biased they are against women's freedom, how frequently they are used to diminish women's status, how commonly—right to this very day—mentioning a woman's period is a means of dismissing or embarrassing her, as demonstrated so publicly by President Trump's remark to Megyn Kelly? Why would women ever invent such a collection of self-defeating ideas?

But the defining of the meaning of menstruation is not just a unilateral action. No matter who initiates any particular myth, stereotype, or misunderstanding, its perpetuation requires wide-scale participation. At the extreme there is a kind of Stockholm Syndrome effect wherein the victim (hostages) of a negative set of values internalize the negatives and then go on to not only live by them but to foist them upon others of the same group. More commonly, the creation of social practices is an interactive endeavor, an organic process in which participants negotiate meaning. When it comes to the social meaning of menstruation, I refer to such engagements as "menstrual transactions," a term meant to encompass social trends in general as well as the day-to-day encounters that individuals have with one another within the larger menstrual ecology. For instance: What are the dynamics when a thirteen-year-old girl buying a box of tampons encounters a male clerk? How do couples decide on what their sexual practices will be during the period and what accommodations do they make? How do boys learn about the menstrual cycle?

It is impossible to know with any certainty why or how men came to view menstruating women and menstrual fluid with fear and disgust, as they so frequently do, although Freud and others have offered provocative speculations regarding ideas such as castration anxiety that deserve consideration. The origins of these prejudices, myths, and superstitions are buried deep within our collective pre-historical pasts. Though their origins are unknown, we do know that powerful menstrual myths can be traced far back into antiquity. We have vivid stories of how male behavior has been shaped by menstrual beliefs. Two of the most striking, and most overlooked, are found in the Bible. One story suggests that male fear of menstruation played a part in the earliest history of the Judeo-Christian faith; the other depicts another male, Jesus Christ himself, as a Menstrual Hero. (See the following chapter for the full discussion.)

There have also been scientific efforts to study aspects of menstrual transactions, including how sexual attraction or desire is affected, in both women and men, by hormonal variations over the course of the phases of the cycle. Using the methodologies of statistical correlation research, one of the most ingenious studies was undertaken in 2007 (Skloot) when a survey was conducted asking women employed as lap dancers to keep track of the stages of their menstrual cycles as well as their income from tips over a two-month period. An analysis of the results that included reports on 5,300 lap dances showed an interaction between cycle phase and hormonal contraception use. Normally cycling participants earned about US$335 per 5-h shift during estrus, US$260 per shift during the luteal phase, and US$185 per shift during menstruation. By contrast, participants using contraceptive pills showed no estrous earnings peak (p. 375).

The implication is that although human females, unlike most other mammals, produce no visible or olfactory indication of being at peak fertility, somehow men become aware of the stage of the cycle, find women more sexually desirable, and reward them accordingly. The hypothesis is yet to be sufficiently validated as to have become part of the canon of reproductive research literature, in part because other hypotheses might explain the outcome. Given the fact that women have learned that many men find menstruation a turn off and, therefore, they try to hide its presence, perhaps the lap dancers who were menstruating tended to hold back from some of the behaviors that were most likely to lead to more generous tipping, regardless of how careful thy were with tampon or cup use so as to guarantee that there was no possible sign of menstrual blood. Although the study should be viewed as inconclusive, it is a good example of efforts to better understand the workings of the menstrual transactions as well as how little is presently understood.

The lengths that women go to in order to keep their periods secret from men is matched only by the lengths men go to in order to avoid knowing about them. I've given a name to this contrived condition: *social amenorrhea*. The word *amenorrhea* is a medical term that means simply "no menstruation." It refers to women who've failed to begin menstruating beyond the customary onset of puberty, or to gymnasts and other athletes and dancers whose diets and physical activities have interfered with their cycles. And it is sometimes a sign of pathology. It's not applied to menopause or pregnancy. *Social amenorrhea* refers to the ways societies and individuals manage to act as though the period doesn't exist.

Women talk about their periods with each other all the time, but in the presence of men they seldom do. Perhaps the best example of this practice is that women needing to change their pad or tampon will invariably carry their entire bag, no matter how cumbersome, to the toilet, rather than risk having a man see them walk through a hall, office, restaurant, or any other public place holding their tampon or pad. Even the design of some handbags reinforces this need with separate zippered compartments for tampon stashing.

Male participation in such subterfuges can be either ignorant or willful. "I don't need to hear this," is a sentence that instructs women to keep their periods to themselves. The shorter version is "Eeew!" Whatever form the message takes, women learn that men don't want to know. Given the fact that, until recently, in any gathering that included a number of women between the ages of 15 and 45, as many as 25% of them are menstruating, it's an achievement that our social arrangements manage to keep the fact hidden. I wrote "until recently" because the rise in the aggressive promotion of menstrual suppression drugs as well as various forms of menstrual activism and the emergence of the transgender movement have the potential to change the menstrual ecology dramatically. The importance of these developments is on a par with the invention of cheap, disposable pads and tampons in the 1920s and '30s and the introduction of birth control pills in the 1960s. Techniques of menstrual cycle management have had profound impacts on both men and women, even though they are used only by women and the relatively small number of transmen who have continued to menstruate.

Male avoidance of menstrual contact requires that women be inculcated with a feeling of repulsion with their own bodies so that they take on the responsibility for protecting men from contamination. Yet, ironically, once women realized that they'd been vested with the magical power of menstrual menace, they figured out how to turn it against their oppressors. A reaction emerged through which the superior strength of the opponent is redirected to defeat him. The process is sometimes called "playing the menstrual card," and assumes many forms, such as the "not tonight, dear" line used to forestall unwanted sexual advances or a woman shyly telling a traffic cop that she ran the stop sign because she was rushing to buy Kotex. An extreme example of a reversal of menstrual power vectors occurred at the Guantanamo Bay military detention facility during the time that it was used to house suspected terrorists who had been captured in Afghanistan or Iraq.

According to transcripts of an FBI investigation into interrogation procedures at the base, part of the psychological technique used to break down the resistance of suspected terrorists was to attack the core of their religious beliefs, thereby presumably making them more vulnerable to revealing the plans and the identities of others. One method was to deface the Quran; another was to deny prisoners the opportunity to practice religious rituals and dietary law. Fundamentalist Islamic ideas about menstruation are Old Testament strict, so a co-ed interrogation team at Git-Mo invented a creative ploy. At one point a woman interrogator reached into her pants and withdrew her hand blotched with red fluid (the record is not clear whether it was actual menstrual blood or fake; another version has her pulling out her bloody tampon) that she smeared on the face of the bound man. This was supposed to show him the powerlessness of his god and the helplessness of his situation. If he didn't tell all he knew, that shameless infidel might daub him yet again with that loathsome matter. Furthermore, since Islamic law required him to cleanse himself of the blood before he could pray or touch his Koran, the water was turned off in his cell (Bonner, 2005, p. A-1). So far, there's been no report on the efficacy of this interrogation method and it hasn't shown up on the list of alleged torture techniques. It isn't specifically covered by the Geneva Conventions unless it falls under the heading of excessive psychological duress.

I consider the Guantanamo "torture" story a good example of a menstrual transaction and a reversal of the usual menstrual rules of order. The parties involved participated (albeit one unwillingly) in an encounter that was based in ancient notions of appropriate menstrual management. However, the woman redefined the meaning of the transaction and the embedded assumptions of power.

Though the Git-Mo incident received some public attention, including mention within a frontpage *New York Times* report on detainee torture, male columnists and opinion writers mostly avoided it. A vociferous condemnation came from Maureen Dowd in a *New York Times* op-ed column titled, "Torture Chicks Gone Wild." Here are some of her comments:

"a toxic combination of sex and religion"

"these missionaries and zealous protectors of values should be worried about the American soul"

"Who are these women? Who allows this to happen? …Why do Rummy and Paul Wolfowitz still have their jobs?"

"Such behavior degrades the women who are doing it …and the country they are doing it for." (2005, p. 17)

Maureen Dowd seems to have adopted the Fundamentalists' point-of-view about the female body. She wrote on a related theme a year later in a column titled, "Who's Hormonal? Hillary or Dick?" (2006, p. A-21). This time she appropriated a common insult that men use against women as well as against other men: accusing the other of menstrually induced instability: "But as the G.O.P. tars Hillary as hysterical, it is important to note that women are affected by lunar tides only once a month, while Dick Cheney has rampaging hormones every day." This is not a new concern for her. Years before the Git-Mo incident Dowd expressed concerns about men blurring the lines of sexual identity. In 1998, in a column titled "Liberties; Pass the Midol" (1998, p. A-25) she fretted about how "men mimic women… to share tender feelings" and ended with the line, "Any minute I'm afraid they might start asking me for Midol."

The female interrogator was hardly the first woman to attack men with her menses. In 1992 during the Reading Music Festival in England a young punk rocker named Donita Sparks and her band L7 were having some technical difficulties that prompted some obnoxious boys in front of the stage to start throwing things at the band. Sparks retaliated by reaching up her skirt, pulling out her tampon and throwing it at the offending audience members, shouting, "Eat my used tampon, fuckers!" The outrageousness of this act parodied the occasional practice of male performers such as James Brown, Willie Nelson, and a long list of others, who commonly throw their sweat soaked handkerchiefs or bandanas to their (female) fans. However, Donita Sparks was performing an act that was both hostile and sexually daring, calculated to gross out the audience, particularly the male members, by flaunting her sexuality in ways far beyond the acceptable.

It is not known if Sparks' transgression of the menstrual norms provoked or quelled the rowdy crowd, but it's unlikely, given male reluctance to come into physical contact with menstrual blood, that anyone threw it back. Instead, I imagine an empty circle forming around the bloody little WMD, a Weapon of Menstrual Destruction, with its fuse-like string, its potential to spread social disorder.

Although there may be less secrecy surrounding the period now than in the past, the subject is still fraught with meaning and anxiety—a constant potential source of tension between men and women, as the following incident that was shared with me reveals. I call it "The Tampon That Broke the Camel's Back." A woman who was in a bad relationship with a man who dominated every aspect of her life seldom left the house. The man did all of the grocery shopping. One day his schedule required that she go to the market. When she came home and they were unpacking the bags, he picked up the box of tampons she had bought and said, "You bought the wrong kind." His presumptuousness suddenly made clear everything that was wrong with the relationship. She divorced him within a year.

The most important characteristic of menstrual etiquette is that men and women both actively maintain the barriers that keep them apart, not only physically but even in a conversational context. Border crossings are tricky under any circumstances, especially when menstrual blood is concerned. Sometimes they are aggressive invasions. At others they can be sweet and loving, as when a man goes out in the rain to buy a woman menstrual products. Menstrual border violations can reveal changes in power relationships at the most profound level, including times of political upheaval. For a brief moment in 1793 the French Revolution was the scene of such a menstrual transaction. On January 21 of that year King Louis XVI was executed and his wife, Queen Marie Antoinette, had been awaiting the tribunal's determination of her fate for nearly nine months. Her supporters hoped that she would be sent into exile, but on October 15 the verdict came down: she too would be sent to the guillotine. The next morning a young gendarme was sent to fetch her. Unfortunately for the Queen, she was menstruating on this fateful day and expected to have enough privacy to change her bloody linens before being taken to the public execution site. But that hope was to be denied. More than thirty years later her chamber attendant, Rosalie Lamorliere, shared the details of what transpired.

> Her majesty passed into the little space between the bed and the wall. . . indicating that I should stand in front of her bed to block the sight of her body from the gendarme. ... The officer instantly approached us and, standing next to the bolster, watched the Queen change. [When she asked for privacy he replied,] "I cannot consent to that," the gendarme responded briskly. "My orders state that I have to keep

an eye on all your movements." ... She carefully rolled up her poor bloody chemise and concealed it in one of her sleeves. ...; then she stuffed that linen into a chink she noticed between the old canvas covering and the wall. (Yalom, 1993, p. 69)

Lest anyone think that men in positions of power presuming the right to intrude in the private realm of menstrual management is rare and isolated to long ago historical anecdotes, consider the following story.

One day in September of 2007, as the new school year was getting off to a start at the Tri-Valley Central High School in Grahamsville, New York, a male security guard crossed the menstrual line. School rules forbade students from carrying their backpacks or other bags into the classroom. According to reports in the local *Times Herald-Record* (Yakin, 2007), as well as more broadly covered in *USA Today* ("Tampon Protests," 2007), a girl was called out of class because she had a small bag and was told that she couldn't carry her purse unless she had her period. The guard then asked, "Do you have your period?"

The girl fled back into her classroom and broke down in tears. In the following days other girls and their parents came forward with similar reports of the guard's intrusive behavior. Soon, the school was in an uproar and protests ensued. Girls wore tampons pinned to their clothing and made purses out of tampon or napkin boxes. In solidarity, and not wanting to be left out of the fun, boys wore maxi-pads stuck to their shirts and one ran through the school naked with a paper bag over his head. A girl who went to speak with the principal wearing a necklace fashioned from a piece of yarn holding an OB tampon box had her tiny talisman confiscated. Parents insisted that the menstrual protocols that protect women from this sort of rude intrusion be rigorously enforced. One mother insisted that, "the school fire these guys." Another demanded, "I don't want him to be able to talk to girls like that," and a father said, "I think serious allegations like this need to be investigated honestly and openly" ("Tampon Protests," 2007).

The incident took on layers of meaning and became a rallying point for girl activism. The details certainly make the guard sound like a creep, or at least an insensitive jerk who, knowingly or not, had abused the authority of his job title and of the power that inhered in him simply because he was an adult male. Had the guard been a woman, the encounter would have passed unnoticed; a female guard would have probably been granted the right to demand that the girl show her a tampon or pad in her purse. The story sounds like a version of the sad menstrual encounter Maria Antoinette endured, and it recapitulates the delineations that are still in place when it comes to menstrual separation.

As just about any woman can testify, when it comes to the period, sisterhood rules. Even women who otherwise would have nothing to do with one another will respond positively to a request for help in avoiding menstrual exposure. An exception to this practice is found in the opening scene of Stephen King's novel, *Carrie* (1974), as well as in film adaptations of the novel (there have been several, as well as theatrical treatments) when the girls in the locker room pelt Carrie (who has just gotten her first period and does not know what is happening) with tampons and pads while screaming at her to "plug it up." Since *Carrie* was written and directed by men, its perspective is skewed. Stephen King (2000) claims he got the idea for the scene when he was a young man of 19 or 20 working with a high school janitor while cleaning the girls' locker room: "There were no urinals, of course, and there were two extra metal boxes on the tile walls—unmarked, and the wrong size for paper towels. I asked what was in them. 'Pussy plugs,' Harry said. 'For them certain days of the month'" (pp. 74–75).

Another popular male novelist who found a way to include a macabre menstrual reference as a plot element was Steig Larsson. In one of the volumes in the Millennium series, *The Girl with the Dragon Tattoo* (2005), Lisbeth Salander and Mikael Blomkvist are discussing the details of a series of murders of women that appear to be linked to religious fanaticism. Salander notes that, "She was tied up and badly abused, but the cause of death was strangulation. She had a sanitary towel down her throat" (p. 375). They go on to conclude that the murder may have been precipitated by the possibility that the victim had violated the Biblical injunction against menstrual sex.

Though men are often depicted as confused or alienated in the presence of menstrual realities, for women menstrual bonding is a common trope; however, it is often played out as a means of demonstrating solidarity against the likelihood of exposure to the humiliating gaze of the mocking male. Even some song lyrics attest to the way women close ranks against men on such occasions. Mary J. Blige's song "PMS" starts out with a direct address to the women in the audience: "I wanna talk to the ladies tonight/ About situation I'm pretty sure y'all be able to relate to/ Trust me." (A full discussion of menstrual music appears in a later chapter.)

A good example of menstrual decorum transgression appears within the sub-culture of the Hells Angels, who've elevated violation of social norms to the top of their gang's ethos. According to Hunter S. Thompson (1966), there are even rewards in the form of jacket patches in the shape of pilot wings for sex acts that are deemed particularly outrageous, "… red wings indicating that the wearer has committed cunnilingus on a menstruating woman, black wings for the same act on a Negress, and brown wings for buggery" (p. 114). In order to qualify for these merit badges (a weird parody of Boy Scout tradition) the act must have been performed in the presence of another member of the gang.

For less extreme examples we find men who have taken upon themselves a responsibility to publicly embrace menstruation as a normal, healthy part of life.

They are men who (not unlike myself) are motivated not just by curiosity but also by a complicated sense of fairness, even gallantry! To coin a phrase, it's a sort of *macho oblige*, a desire to make a contribution to gender equality by demonstrating to the world that a mature, liberated man is capable of being at ease with the period.

Consider the work of Harry Finley. Founder and curator of the Museum of Menstruation and Women's Health, Finley is a man who might best be described as a menstrual hobbyist, an amateur collector who, in 1995, opened, in the basement of his home in New Carrollton, Maryland, a suburb of Washington, D.C., a display of menstrual paraphernalia, including belts, pads, cups, sponges, tampons, and other products as well as booklets, videos, magazines and advertisements—all pertaining to the cultural history of menstruation. His web site (www.mum.org) is an impressive collection of information covering such topics as menstrual art and poetry, essays, history, video sources, and product manufacturer references. It is probably the best starting location for anyone setting out to research any aspect of the topic.

The question commonly asked of Finley's enterprise is, "Why would a man collect stuff having to do with menstruation?" The question is *not*, "Why would *anyone* collect that stuff?" It is a gendered question and carries with it the implication that menstruation is off limits to men. According to Karen Houppert, who interviewed him for her book *The Curse* (1999), Finley himself seems clueless about his own motivation other than to say that he finds the subject interesting (pp. 210–213). Finley is aware of the fact that his interest makes him an object of curiosity or even ridicule, particularly because he has no background in curatorial studies, museum management, or any other pertinent field. His answer, posted on his web site, suggests that he sees his creation as an expression of his own courageous personality:

> What qualifies me is having had the nerve to create it, buttressed by my interest in the cultural history of menstruation... Before I started MuM, I had to decide if I wanted to suffer the criticism it would of course bring; the enterprise had to be good. I've had no reason to regret my MuM. (2018)

If Harry Finley is at one end of the menstrual sensitivity scale, most men can be found somewhere in the middle. I once witnessed the full spectrum of male views of menstrual etiquette at a social gathering of eight men at a friend's apartment. There had been a fair amount of drinking and smoking as we relaxed and got to know one another. The host mentioned that his wife had recently remodeled the apartment, and some of the chairs were upholstered in a rich, white fabric. I asked the other men to tell me how they would react if there were a party going on and they saw a woman get up from one of the white chairs leaving behind a large red stain. I was surprised at how quickly several men responded. The first said sternly, "I'd call her on it!" When someone asked what he meant, he became irate, "She should know when she's getting it. There's no reason to be unprepared. That's disgusting!" The second man said he'd tell another woman about it so she wouldn't have the embarrassment of thinking that the men knew. A third said he'd discretely cover the stain with a napkin so others wouldn't notice. A fourth laughed as he got up and enacted how he would walk closely behind her in a kind of clown stride so no one would see as he escorted her to the bathroom. The host just shook his head and sighed, "My wife would kill her."

The tone of the conversation was part goofy and part angry, and several men were dumbfounded by the question. They had no idea what they would do other than act as though nothing had happened, or at least nothing that required their intervention. It seemed to me that this small sample of responses covered nearly the full range of possibilities, from gallantry to hostility, with bewilderment settled in the middle.

A few years ago I was subjected to an actual test of menstrual etiquette. I'd given a colleague a ride home after an evening's professional/social event, and, as she got out of my car, I noticed something dark on the beige seat of the car. At first I thought she'd dropped something out of her bag, and I called to her. But then I noticed that it was a stain and that her dress was soiled as well. I quickly covered the mark with my hand and said goodnight. I don't know if she noticed, or, if when she got home, she wondered if she'd bled on the seat, but neither of us mentioned it when we saw each other at work the next day. When I got home, I told my wife what had happened and returned to the car with water and rags to clean the mark. It turns out that just as women have been conditioned to feel embarrassed if a man knows they're menstruating, men have also been conditioned to feel embarrassed if they accidentally notice evidence of the period.

When and how does the conditioning of male ignorance and avoidance begin? Like so many other aspects of our conditioning, the home and schools are the two chief influences. Consider the implications of health education in the schools.

Although health and sex education curricula have changed over the nearly 80 years since the earliest efforts to introduce these subjects into the school curriculum, they continue to have a few common characteristics that have changed little. In spite of efforts in more "progressive" schools to educate boys and girls together about the human body, programs are still more commonly segregated when it comes to menstrual education. (I'm referring here to practices within the United States. Elsewhere, particularly in Sweden and many other European countries, classes are fully gender integrated.) Here we see, once again, the value of Marshall McLuhan's sage aphorism, "The Medium Is the Message." What do boys and girls learn by the fact that they are shepherded into separate rooms for "the talk?"

The two most important elements have nothing to do with the content of the lessons. First is the fact that it's deemed inappropriate for boys and girls to learn about this sex stuff together, unlike every other subject in the curriculum. Even gym and shop classes are now gender integrated in many schools! An air of mystery and forbidden knowledge is created by the separation. Even though the lessons strive to teach girls to feel positive about their bodies, even proud of their newly acquired reproductive potential, the fact that the classes have an air of secrecy undermines the good intentions. Why would you hide from boys unless you thought they'd make fun of you if they knew what you were learning about? Why would you shut the boys out unless you felt there might be something shameful about what you were doing?

For boys, the feeling of otherness is enhanced by the differences in the hygiene kits that each group usually receives. The deodorants, soaps or razors in the male packages are far less gender coded than the pads or tampons in the "starter kits" for the girls. Furthermore, as Karen Houppert points out in *The Curse* (1999), the emphasis on hygiene rather than sex and reproduction that dominates menstrual education reinforces the impression that the period is somehow dirty. And yet, even as a hygienic concern, the period must be denied. Houppert states the case well:

> People with runny noses do not hide their tissues from colleagues and family members. They do not die of embarrassment when they sneeze in public. Young girls do not cringe if a boy spies them buying a box of Kleenex. Caught without a hanky on a cold day, people sometimes use their sleeves; they are sheepish but not humiliated. They do not blush or stammer or hide the evidence. No one celebrates congestion. It is inconvenient and occasionally, when accompanied by a cold, decidedly unpleasant. But those who suffer publicly—*ah-choo!*—are casually blessed. It is, in essence, no big deal. The same is not true of periods. (p. 4)

The second "lesson" in the way the education is structured is embedded in the fact that the classes are always taught by a member of the same sex as the students. Men talk to boys, and women talk to girls, in the belief that the kids will be more comfortable hearing the facts from one of their own. Of course, the arrangement merely reinforces the idea that the content is restricted to one's gender. If the school authorities believe, as their instructional arrangements clearly suggest, that information concerning sexuality, particularly the menstrual cycle, can only be purveyed by a member of one's own sex, then how can we expect boys and girls to feel they could or should be comfortable talking to each other easily about their bodies and their feelings about their bodies?

Although sex education curricula do cover reproductive biology, good hygiene, good manners, and respect for others, they also inadvertently tend to leave boys with the feeling that girls are mysterious beings whose bodies are shrouded in secrecy, and that boys should refrain from expressing curiosity about menstruation out of respect for girls' embarrassment. An example of this state of affairs was expressed by a woman who told me of a twelve-year-old boy who asked her, "Why don't they just hold it until they get to the bathroom?" His expectation that girls could be "toilet trained" as he was encapsulates the kinds of misunderstandings that boys grow up with and that most eventually unlearn, though there is no guarantee that all men do.

Every culture, every generation, and every individual is the recipient of a body of menstrual lore that shapes male values, beliefs and behavior. At the same time, every culture, every generation, and every individual participates in reshaping menstrual meanings through the transactions they engage in. Ushered in by a combination of a new generation of menstrual activists, legislative initiatives focused on removing sales taxes on menstrual products and improved regulation of product content, a new generation of cycle management pharmaceuticals and, perhaps most notably, the movement to broaden the fundamental definitions of gender resulting from the trans-gender movement, we are now entering a new era of menstrual relations, a "Post-Menstrual Age" that will challenge all of the social practices that have been layered upon the biology of the menstrual cycle. It remains to be seen what gains and losses the changes will yield.

References

Bonner, R. (2005, February 13). Detainee says he was tortured in U.S. custody. *New York Times*, p. A-1.

Dowd, M. (1998, April 15). Liberties: Pass the Midol. *New York Times*, p. A-25.

Dowd, M. (2005, January 30). Torture chicks gone wild. *New York Times*, p. WK-17.

Dowd, M. (2006, February 8). Who's hormonal? Hillary or Dick? *New York Times*, p. A-21.

Evans, J., & Read, S. (2017). *Maladies & medicine: Exploring health & healing, 1540–1740*. South Yorkshire, England: Pen & Sword Books.

Finley, H. Retrieved June 2, 2018, from http://www.mum.org/

Frick, A. (2009, May 29). G. Gordon Liddy on Sotomayor: "Let's hope that key conferences aren't when she's menstruating." *Think Progress*. Retrieved June 2, 2018, from https://thinkprogress.org/g-gordon-liddy-on-sotomayor-lets-hope-that-the-key-conferences-aren-t-when-she-s-menstruating-2f571da16641/

Houppert, K. (1999). *The curse: Confronting the last unmentionable taboo: menstruation.* New York, NY: Farrar, Straus and Giroux.

King, S. (2000). *On writing: A memoir of the craft.* New York, NY: Scribners.

Larsson, S. (2005). *The girl with the dragon tattoo.* New York, NY: Alfred A. Knopf.

Levi, C. (1947). *Christ stopped at Eboli.* New York, NY: Farrar, Straus and Giroux.

Mulvey-Roberts, M. (2003, February 24). *Menstrual mythologies.* Keynote Address presented at Menstruation: Blood, Body, Brand. University of Liverpool, Liverpool, England.

Qaddafi, M. (n.d.). *The green book.* Retrieved June 12, 2018, from http://www.911-truth.net/other-books/Muammar-Qaddafi-Green-Book-Eng.pdf

Rucker, P. (2015, August 8). Trump says Fox's Megyn Kelly had "blood coming out of her wherever." *The Washington Post.* Retrieved June 2, 2018, from https://www.washingtonpost.com/news/post-politics/wp/2015/08/07/trump-says-foxs-megyn-kelly-had-blood-coming-out-of-her-wherever/?noredirect=on&utm_term=.f81f4ae4dbae

Shlain, L. (2003). *Sex, time, and power: How women's sexuality shaped human evolution.* New York, NY: Viking Press.

Skloot, R. (2007, December 9). Lap-Dance science. *New York Times.* Retrieved July 3, 2017 from https://www.nytimes.com/2007/12/09/magazine/09lapdance.html

Tampon Protests Distract N.Y. School. (2007, September 28). *Newsok.* Retrieved from https://newsok.com/article/3136562/tampon-protests-distract-ny-school

Thompson, H. (1966). *Hell's angels: A strange and terrible saga.* New York, NY: Ballantine Books.

Yakin, H. (2007, September 28). "The Question" causes furor at local high school. *Times Herald-Record.*

Yalom, M. (1993). *Blood sisters: The French revolution in women's memory.* New York, NY: Pandora.

CHAPTER TWO

Blood in the Bible, Torah, and Quran and How Jesus Became a Menstrual Hero

What if men and boys were required to take a bath every time they masturbated, had a wet dream or an orgasm? What if any time their pants had a drop of semen on them they had to be washed? Well, that's just what the ancient Biblical scriptures required of men, virtually the same kinds of requirements as for women regarding their menstrual fluid. But somehow the rules for men have been generally ignored while those for women continued to have considerable impact across cultures and centuries. Otherwise, imagine the hordes of adolescent boys lined up each morning at the ritual bath and the throngs of men impatiently checking their cell phones while awaiting their turns to be cleansed. Consider the impact if the rules laid down in Leviticus 15:16–19 were widely obeyed:

> When a man has an emission of semen, he must bathe his whole body with water, and he will be unclean till evening. Any clothing or leather that has semen on it must be washed with water, and it will be unclean till evening. When a man has sexual relations with a woman and there is an emission of semen, both of them must bathe with water, and they will be unclean till evening. When a woman has her regular flow of blood, the impurity of her monthly period will last seven days, and anyone who touches her will be unclean till evening. (New International Version)

While seminal fluid certainly has its own symbolic power, it has not been as thoroughly codified and ritualized as menses with its huge array of euphemisms, taboos, products, industries, ad campaigns, and culturally inscribed beliefs. As the three Abrahamic faiths evolved, each one developed unique rules, rituals, practices, and lore pertaining to menstrual management. Jewish customs, for example, became thoroughly articulated with precisely codified guidelines under the heading of *niddah*, the term used to refer to a menstruating woman which translates as "in a state of pollution." The cleansing practice even came to include an architectural feature, the *mikveh*, a specific location or building dedicated to the performance of a cleansing bath following the end of menstruation that prepared women to return to sexual relations with their husbands during the phase of the menstrual cycle when ovulation, and thus conception, are most likely. Modern *mikveh* practice has been broadened to include other symbolic cleansing and transitional rituals, but the basic link to post-menstrual preparation for sexual congress still prevails.

Jewish menstrual rules of order have been codified over the centuries. For instance, Moses Maimonides (1135–1204) claimed that menstruating women were not sexually attractive, placing them in the same category as those who are elderly or menopausal (Brozyna, 2005, p. 163). Similarly, the *Midrash Rabbah*, a foundational document of Hebrew Scripture, contended that children born with leprosy were the result of women having intercourse while they were menstruating (Brozyna, 2005, p. 253).

Building upon the Leviticus prohibitions, Islam also constructed a set of beliefs surrounding the menstrual cycle. Most are found in the Koran and other texts that are said to be accounts of statements or acts performed by Muhammad or one of his contemporaries. For instance, the 114 chapters of the *Koran* are known as *suras*, and *sura* number 2.222 states,

> And they ask you about menstruation. Say: It is a discomfort; therefore keep aloof from the women during the menstrual discharge and do not go near them until they have become clean; then when they have cleansed themselves, go in to them as Allah has commanded you…. (Brozyna, 2005, p. 284)

(Note: some English translations use the term "illness" rather than "discomfort," a good example of the difficulty of discerning the nuances of meaning in ancient texts.)

One of the most interesting ways that Islam diverges from its fellow faiths is the inclusion of women's perspectives on a number of matters, though reports of their views were written by men. Several Hadiths, stories about Muhammad and his contemporaries, include a woman's first-person account of her menstrual experiences, including one about an embarrassing experience of getting a first period while riding a camel and staining the saddle (Brozyna, 2005, p. 289). Another woman reported that the Prophet would sleep with a menstruating wife but avoid having sex with her. An indication of how nuanced some of the interpretations of the sexual protocols were is captured in the writings of an Islamic theologian, Abu Hamid al-Ghazali (1058–1128), in a text titled *Book on the Etiquette of Marriage* (Brozyna, 2005, p. 289). After reinforcing the "no menstrual sex" rule, he goes on to discuss alternative activities and suggests that it is permissible for a wife to masturbate her husband and for him to continue to sleep with her, though sodomy is also to be avoided.

Underlying this rich accumulation of religious lore with all its subtle variations and accretions of meaning, there lurk several core questions: why did men make up all these rules and beliefs in the first place? What were they trying to control and explain? Perhaps the creators of the Leviticus restrictions had gained a remarkable insight into the biological workings of the female reproductive system. The human animal is almost unique in the fact that its sexual appetite is unrelated to its ovulatory cycle. Humans can be aroused at any moment, regardless of whether the act is likely to result in pregnancy. Almost all other animals are aroused to sexual desire when triggered by the visual and olfactory signals given off by the ovulating females. Somehow humans figured out that, from the point-of-view of species perpetuation, there was little point in having intercourse during the flow of blood, but that doing so during the week following had a good chance of leading to insemination. Furthermore, given the fact that delaying the fulfillment of sexual pleasure enhanced sexual desire, creating cultural prohibitions against sexual contact during non-productive periods had a positive effect on increasing pregnancy rates.

Probably the most challenging aspect of the menstrual phenomenon is that menstrual blood so closely resembles arterial blood. And men have likely been confounded by the similarity since prehistoric times. After all, the human species is nearly unique with it comes to having a menstrual cycle. As Shlain (2003) points out, of the approximately 4,000 species of mammals, very few experience a regular blood loss. In fact, of the nearly 270 different species of primates, only 31 of those species menstruate (p. 17).

To make matters even more confusing, there is widespread ignorance regarding the differences between the vaginal secretion associated with *estrus* (the period of fertility) and the secretion that accompanies the shedding of the uterine lining, *menses*. People commonly believe that the show of blood their pet female dog displays means that, "Fifi is getting her period." In fact, it's the opposite. A show of vaginal blood in a dog or other mammal means that it is ovulating; it is in heat and at the height of fertility. In a human female a show of blood indicates that the individual is at her lowest likelihood of conceiving, is not presently ovulating.

Furthermore, human mammals practice concealed ovulation; there are no signals alerting the males of the species that this is a good time to copulate. The human species is nearly alone in not having a distinct period of estrus but, rather, is prone to engage in intercourse at any time during the menstrual cycle, regardless of whether or not ovulation is occurring. In effect, in humans a vaginal discharge indicates that there's no point in copulation (other than for pleasure!) because conception is unlikely (though not impossible). In other animals it's the ideal time since fertility is at its peak.

Early male confusion must have been profound. Much of what humans learned about biology surely came from observing the behavior of other species, including copulation, birthing, and other reproductive behaviors. But humans do it all differently. They do not have a "mating season" as they are always ready to rut. Furthermore, female humans far outlive their reproductive capacity; other animals ovulate for their entire life spans. Human females nurse and care for their young for years before an infant can fend for itself; other mammals seldom require more than a few months or even less before a high degree of self sufficiency is attained.

But what does all this have to do with how the ancient scriptures set about encoding views on the menstrual cycle? There are very few menstrual references in the *Bible* itself, other than the previously cited set of rules and one that uses a reference to menses as a means of describing the human condition as filthy and disgusting, though not all translations are as explicit as this one from the 1899 Douay-Rheims version:

> And we are all become as one unclean, and all our justices as the rag of a menstruous woman: and we have all fallen as a leaf, and our iniquities, like the wind, have taken us away. (Isaiah 64:5)

It is impossible to know with any certainty how men came to view menstruating women and menstrual fluid with fear and disgust, as they so frequently have. The origins of these prejudices, myths, and superstitions are buried deep within our collective pre-historical pasts. One way of delving into the ways that the beliefs or superstitions actually affected the lives of the people is to examine the rare specific stories of menstrual transactions, incidents when men and women had to live up to (or violate) the rigid codes of behavior. There are three such stories in the Bible.

One story suggests that male fear of menstruation played a part in the earliest history of the Judeo-Christian faith. Another suggests that ignoring the menstrual messages the body sends can lead to disaster. The third depicts Jesus Christ himself as a Menstrual Hero.

If Sigmund Freud had been a woman and a Biblical scholar, perhaps we'd not be so familiar with Sophocles' story of Oedipus, the tale of a man's bizarre and twisted relationships with his mother and father, but instead we'd be more familiar with Rachel's story in the Old Testament book of Genesis. The story of Rachel is one of the most powerful narratives of a father-daughter encounter in Western literature, surely as psychologically profound as that of Oedipus or of King Lear and his three daughters. Rather than Sophocles' story of the male child rising up to strike down the parent of the same sex, Genesis tells a story of a woman employing the very element that was thought to make her weak and soiled, her menstrual blood, as a weapon to vanquish the overbearing, abusive and hated father. It is contained in less than 20 brief verses of Genesis 31, yet it encapsulates one of the fundamental aspects of gender relationships.

The background to the story is that Jacob had married Rachel, daughter of Laban, an Old Testament despot, and agreed to work for Laban tending his flocks. After twenty years Jacob felt he'd paid all of his debts to Laban, who'd been a harsh, demanding taskmaster to both Jacob and Rachel. One day while Laban was away in the hills tending his sheep, Jacob decided to take his extensive family, his servants, his sheep, and his belongings and return to his home in Canaan. In order to get even with her father for all the years of abuse she suffered, Rachel slipped into Laban's tent before they left and stole his collection of household gods, or *teraphim*, and took them away with her.

When Laban returned from the hills and found out what happened, he set off in pursuit of Jacob and his entourage, eventually catching up with them in the hills of Gilead where he berated Jacob for sneaking off and accused him of stealing his *teraphim*, which he believed to be sources of power and protection from evil. Jacob denied that anyone in his camp had taken the objects, invited Laban to search wherever he liked, and promised to kill whoever was found with them. Laban searched thoroughly, coming to Rachel's tent last, as good drama requires. He ransacked the tent, feeling around in every bag, sack, and hanging. Finally, the only place he hadn't looked was under the camel saddle and blankets that Rachel was sitting on. As he approached her, she tried a desperate ploy—or perhaps it was simply an *ancient* ploy, one older, and more reliable than history can possible recount.

Consider the challenge faced by those theologians, Biblical scholars, and compilers of the Torah who had the task of interpreting its meaning or of translating the text into English. They had to deal with the same kinds of restrictions and sensitivity surrounding mention of menstruation in their own cultures, centuries after the original text was recorded. Note the evasions and euphemisms they employed. It is impossible to know to what extent they accurately capture the semantic practices of the ancient times or if they are reflections of the requirements of the translators' day and age:

> "And she said to her father, let it not displease my lord that I cannot rise up before thee; for the custom of women is upon me." (King James Version)
>
> "Let not my lord be angry that I cannot rise before you, for the way of women is upon me." (Revised Standard Version)
>
> "Rachel said to her father, 'Do not take it amiss, sir, that I cannot rise in your presence: the common lot of woman is upon me.'" (The New English Bible)
>
> "Rachel said to her father, 'Let not my lord feel offended that I cannot rise in your presence; a woman's period is upon me.'" (The Catholic Study Bible)
>
> "For she said to her father, 'Let not my father take it amiss that I cannot rise before you, for the period of women is upon me.'" (The Torah: A Modern Commentary)

Consider the dramatic—even cinematic!—qualities of this moment. Rachel has told her father that she has her period and cannot stand up out of respect for him because she is bleeding. Laban stops cold. At first he may have been shocked just by the fact that a daughter would dare to mention menstruation to her father, even if she used the most polite and subtle of euphemisms. Then, the implications of her statement dawn on him. The menstrual rules of order were clear, as spelled out in the verses from Leviticus: "When a woman has a discharge of blood from her body, she shall be in her impurity for seven days, and whoever touches her shall be unclean until the evening."

If Laban touches Rachel or the objects that she is sitting on, he will be contaminated and shunned by the men gathered outside until he has gone through the required cleansing rituals. Everyone will witness his degradation. To make matters worse, Laban's uncleanness would have come from the menstrual blood of his own daughter, giving the violation an extra taint of incestuous contact. And if in fact the icons are under Rachel and she has bled on them, they'd have been defiled and rendered useless to him; he'd be unable to take them home anyway and the cost of locating the now worthless items would include his own debasement.

Imagine the tension as father and daughter stare at one another, she in defiance, he in doubt of her honesty. He's certain that she's stolen his icons and has them hidden under her, but he can't tell if she's lying about her period. Furthermore, he can't go to Jacob for help with his investigation because of the humiliation he'd suffer at having been defeated by a woman—worse yet, his daughter. The suspense is resolved when Laban accepts his loss, turns his back on his daughter forever, and storms out of the tent. But he must do something to save face, particularly with the men who've been awaiting the outcome of his search. His solution is almost comical in light of the way modern readers have been trained to read Freudian significance into certain physical objects: Laban rushes out to build a stone phallus, a pillar that will mark the new boundaries between Laban's land and that which has been ceded to Jacob. What's more, he gets Rachel's husband and the other men in his camp to help him construct the erection, invoking a spirit of male solidarity while attempting to create a manifestation of his power that has a permanence beyond that of his daughter's (and all women's) monthly days of freedom from male control:

> Then Laban ... said to Jacob, ... "Come now, let us make a covenant, you and I; and let it be a witness between you and me." So Jacob took a stone, and set it up as a pillar. And Jacob said to his kinsmen, "Gather stones," and they took stones, and make a heap; and they ate by the heap. (Genesis 31: 44–46, Revised Standard Version)

Though Laban and Jacob go on to build stone markers to differentiate their respective territories, it seems as though Laban is equally motivated by a desire to wall out his daughter and her unanticipated assertiveness in wielding her menstrual blood as a weapon against her father. The story leaves little doubt that Laban has been beaten and emasculated; he has lost both his possessions and his power.

This story is a significant marker in the epic saga of human menstrual relations and warrants more attention than it has received, though there have been some noteworthy observations. Among the more interesting is Nahum Sarna's (1996) comment:

> ... it is not at all improbable that to the narrator the culminating absurdity in the religious situation was reached when Rachel hid the idols in the camel cushion and sat upon them in a state of menstrual impurity. In the light of the Israelite notions of the clean and unclean, the description of Rachel's act implies an attitude of willful defilement and scornful rejection of their religious significance. (p. 201)

The most radical interpretation of the incident might claim that Rachel's use of her menstrual blood to contaminate Laban's gods was an early blow against polytheistic religions and an opening to the monotheistic beliefs that emerged in the ensuing years. But, to the best of my knowledge, that proposition has not yet gained traction.

There is another menstrual conundrum in the dissemination of this story: how can paintings, book illuminations, and other image media represent the confrontation between father and daughter in all its dramatic elements yet avoid any explicit details that depict the presence of menstrual reality? In fact, Laban's fruitless search for his stolen icons became a very popular subject for painters with versions being created by Antonio Belucci (Italian, 1654–1726), Francesco Fernandl (Italian, 1679–1740), Giovanna Battista Tiepolo (Italian, 1726–1729), Francesco

Zugno (Italian, 1708–1787), Pieter Lastman (Dutch, 1583–1633), Willem van Nieulandt (Dutch, 1584–1635), Pietro da Cortona (Italian, 1596–1669), Laurent de la Hyre (French, 1606–1656), Bartolome Esteban Murillo (Spanish, 16161–1682), Jan Victors (Dutch, 1620–1676), and Hendrik Heerschop (Dutch (1620–1672), to name just a few.

In retelling the tale on canvas all of the artists have taken liberties with the details. For instance, it is clearly implied in the text that Laban went through the tents searching for his possessions alone while Jacob and his followers waited outside. But in virtually every one of the paintings Laban and Rachel are surrounded by an observing crowd as he opens a trunk, peers behind curtains or stares at Rachel who reclines atop her camel saddle. His futile search is witnesses by many.

Renditions of the encounter in illuminated manuscripts are similarly dramatized. The only suggestion in the pictures of a menstrual presence is the fact that Rachel is often seen sprawled across a red blanket or rug or there is some other red fabric near her. Sometimes she is wearing a red garment. Such details are both subtle and effective, especially for any observer already familiar with the elements of the text itself. In the Morgan Library collection of manuscripts there is one especially amusing and heavily freighted illumination (Weltchronik, 1360). It depicts a blond-haired Rachel seated at the opening of her small tent while Laban and one of his men stand facing her. She has her right hand raised while her left tries to push back into the tent a red faced, goat-like animal with a long horn. It appears that the anonymous illustrator charged with the job of rendering the moment had his own notions of how the menstrual cycle might affect a woman's demeanor, including the idea that women on their periods were possessed by dangerous animal qualities that should be avoided.

As mentioned, despite its high drama, so full of deep cultural and psychological nuances, the parent-child confrontation told in this arresting tale has received scant attention by theologians, cultural anthropologists, literary scholars and a host of others one might have expected to have delved into its layers of meaning. What would it say about our cultural landscape today if this tale had risen to a place of prominence in our shared mythos? Would we speak of men with an inordinate fear of menstrual blood or fear of women in general as having a "Rachel Complex," or of mean-willed, spirit-breaking fathers, particularly fathers of girls, as "Labanites?"

Regardless of the relative scarcity of menstrual legends, there does exist in the collective mythos a body of beliefs and practices that entail many nuances of the Rachel and Laban story. From childhood through old age, boys and girls, men and women engage in acts that reflect notions of what defines the appropriate menstrual relationship. It seems that menstrual management is among the central organizing concerns of human behavior at both the social and personal level; the way menstrual transactions are managed encapsulates all of the social assumptions about gender separation and difference.

And though neither Sophocles nor Freud nor any other widely recognized writer or dramatist has risen to the challenge of placing menstrual power at the center of collective consciousness, the power that Rachel employed is understood by every high school girl who has ever instinctively followed Rachel's lead to get out of gym class.

The love story of Rachel and Jacob is one of the central chronicles in Biblical studies. Testimony to its influence is found, in fact, in the popularity of their names. But, the incidents surrounding Rachel's theft of her father's *teraphim* and the role that the menstrual taboos played in her escaping punishment receive little attention. Until, that it, the publication in 1997 of Anita Diamant's *The Red Tent.*

Diamant's novel employs a hybrid literary genre that involves selecting a secondary character in a well-known work and retelling the story from that character's perspective. John Updike's retelling of *Hamlet* in *Gertrude and Claudius* (2000) is a good example of the technique.

The Red Tent is told in the first person by a character named Dinah, a daughter of Leah and Jacob, who narrates her life story with emphasis on the lives of the women in the extended family. The title refers to the special tent that is erected for women to stay in during their periods as well as for childbirth and any other aspect of life having to do with women's reproductive processes. The novel was a best seller, has been published in more than 25 countries, and was adapted as a two-part, four-hour miniseries for TV. The success of the book even enabled Diamant to establish a modern version of the *mikveh*, the ritual Jewish immersion bath facility, near Boston.

Like all such creations in this category of derivative fiction, the novel sometimes takes sweeping liberties with its source material, adding characters and subplots, fleshing out social and psychological influences, embellishing descriptions of settings, and enriching character relationships. In dong so the original, concise details in Genesis that span barely a dozen pages are expanded into a book of more than 300 pages in length. Among the most striking are those concerning the menstrual showdown.

While the details in Genesis of Laban's attempt to recover his missing *teraphim* are sparse, the text leaves the impression that he was not sure that Rachel was hiding them under her blankets and that she had her period. It is clear, though, that he was unwilling to risk being soiled by possible contact. The text also presents Rachel as a daughter who, though she has good reason to resent her father, still shows him respect while she denies having stolen his gods. Diamant turns all of these elements upside down.

The confrontation scene comes after a long sequence describing the trek that Jacob's entourage was undertaking. And the fact that Laban was able to catch up with them is due in part to the fact that they had to pause for three days to erect the red tent to accommodate the onset of the women's periods. When charged with theft, Jacob adamantly denied the charge, invited Laban to search their encampment and then stormed off into the woods. The search proceeds:

> After Laban had ransacked my father's tent, there was nowhere left for him to search except the red tent. His eyes fixed upon the women's tent on the edge of the camp. It was unthinkable that a healthy man would walk of his own will inside that place during the head of the month. The men and boys stared to see if he would place himself among bleeding women-even worse, his own daughters.

Laban hesitates for a moment but decides to defy the taboos. He enters the tent and is about to dig through the pile of blankets, but at this point the action takes a turn:

> Rachel stood up from her place on the straw. She did not drop her eyes as she addressed her father. Indeed, she stared straight into his face, and without anger or fear or any apparent emotion she said, "I took them, Father. I have all of the *teraphim*. All of your gods. They are here. I sit upon them. The *teraphim* of our family now bathe in my monthly blood, by which your household gods are polluted beyond redemption. You can have them if you wish," Rachel continued calmly, as though she were speaking of trifling things. "I will dig them out and even wipe them off for you if you like, father, but their magic has been turned against you. You are without their protection from this time forward." (Diamant, 1997, pp. 117–118)

This description inverts what we might call the "passive aggressive" behavior of the Rachel of Genesis who is demure in her apology to her father for not respecting his presence by standing as she should. In the retelling, Rachel is fully assertive as she plays the strongest weapon she has, the polluting power of her menstrual blood. Not only does she blatantly confess her crime, she revels in it by telling him that his gods "now bathe in my monthly blood," and that she'd be glad to return them to him if he'd like her to "wipe them off for you" (p. 118). Were he to accept the offer it would be an even greater humiliation. And there is no question that she actually does have her period as the moment takes place within the red tent that was erected for the purpose of giving the women a sanctified place to go away from the men.

Upon Laban's departure from the tent he must still deal with Jacob and the other men waiting outside. In order to save face he says nothing about Rachel's defiance and acts as though it was a failed search. To mend fences he proposes to Jacob that they build "a cairn to mark the boundaries between them" (p. 118). Then, as in the original story, the men go up into the hills to pile up stones in a symbolic gesture to reassert their manly power.

In the Bible there is no further mention of Laban or of his stolen *teraphim*, but Anita Diamant reintroduces the objects 50 pages and about 8 years later in Dinah's narration once Jacob and his followers arrive in Cannan. As the story line required, the occurrence of Dinah's first period is an important development, not only for her but as a way of revealing more aspects of the lives of women and the menstrual rituals that take place in the sanctuary of the red tent. Dinah's menarche leads to a description of an event called "the ceremony for opening the womb" (p. 174).

When Dinah informed Rachel and the other women that she had begun to bleed, they immediately began to celebrate with dancing and feasting, as well as having her repeatedly drink a strong wine from a special metal cup. They put Kohl on her eye, perfume her body, and see that she gets quite drunk, "My mother kept my wine cup filled and brought it to my lips so often that soon I found it difficult to speak..." (p. 171). Then, to her surprise, Rachel brings out the *teraphim* she had stolen from Laban and selects one:

> ... the goddess wearing the shape of a grinning frog. Her wide mouth held her own eggs for safekeeping, while her legs were splayed in a dagger shaped triangle, ready to lay a thousand more. Rachel rubbed the obsidian figure with oil until the creature gleamed and dripped in the light of the lamps. I stared at the frog's silly face and giggled, but no one laughed with me. (p. 172)

The girl is stripped of her robe and the women take her outside the tent into the night where they place her face down on hands and knees with arms outstretched. The women surround her and Rachel performs the ritual:

> It did not hurt. The oil eased the entry, and the narrow triangle fit perfectly as it entered me. I faced the west while the little goddess faced east as she broke the lock of my womb. When I cried out, it was not so much pain but surprise and perhaps even pleasure, for it seemed to me that the Queen herself was lying on top of me, with Dumuzi her consort beneath me. (pp. 172–173)

It's hard to imagine a more radical reconstruction of Biblical lore. The scene expresses vividly the larger message of the book, that the familiar tales, written by men, featuring men, interpreted by men and perpetuated by men, would have completely different meanings—even contrary meanings—if told by and about women. These tales, after all, are written and repeated in the interest of those who wrote them. They are not merely fanciful anecdotes shared around a campfire and then set aside in the light of day. And in the case of menstrual–themed tales such as that of Rachel and Laban or those expressed in contemporary jokes or insults, their purpose is one of reinforcement of social roles and rules of order. The value of Anita Diamant's retelling lies in its willingness to reframe an ancient way of seeing and, thereby, suggest a reconsideration of contemporary practices and beliefs.

Now consider yet another aspect of how the Bible used the menstrual cycle to dramatic effect. There is only one other Old Testament story involving the menstrual cycle, a tale that describes the corruption of a king and, years later, led to the creation of a high–class form of Biblical pornography, the story of King David and Bathsheba.

The second book of Samuel depicts the lechery of the king and his plot to kill the husband of the woman he has debauched:

> And it came to pass in an eveningtide, that David arose from off his bed, and walked upon the roof of the king's house: and from the roof he saw a woman washing herself; and the woman was very beautiful to look upon. And David sent and enquired after the woman. And one said, Is not this Bathsheba, the daughter of Eliam, the wife of Uriah the Hittite? And David sent messengers, and took her; and she came in unto him, and he lay with her; for she was purified from her uncleanness: and she returned unto her house. And the woman conceived, and sent and told David, and said, I am with child. (2 Samuel 11: 1–5 King James Version)

It turns out that Bathsheba was having her post-menstrual bath; David may have observed her at the equivalence of a *mikveh*. This is the significance of the reference to her having been "purified from her uncleanness," indicating that she was entering the segment of her menstrual cycle when she was most likely to be ovulating and, therefore, most likely to conceive, which is exactly what happened. In this case, the prohibition against menstrual sex worked just as it was supposed to except that the consequences were catastrophic. Not only did she get pregnant, but due to the fact that her husband was away at war, it would be clear to the community that the conception was the result of adultery. King David tried to finesse the situation by urging Bathsheba's husband, Uriah, to go home and sleep with his wife, but he choose instead to stay with his men who were on leave from the battle front. The drama heightens when David, now desperate to hide his sin, sends orders that Uriah is to be placed at the front of the battle lines so that he will be killed and people will assume that the child his wife will bear was his.

This is the earliest known example of the use of a missed period for dramatic effect as a plot device. It is the predecessor of thousands that followed which are frequently introduced with the simple sentence, "I'm late," some form of which is exactly what Bathsheba's message to David stated. The moral of the story is presumably that adultery is a sin and can lead to the downfall of even so great a man as King David; however, the story has also been interpreted in such a way as to depict Bathsheba as a temptress, a wily slut who used her body to tempt the virtuous king into a liaison that gave her a place in the palace at the expense of her virtuous husband.

While the general view expressed in exegeses from medieval times to the present has been that Bathsheba was taking a post-menstrual bath, there is one noteworthy—and even kinky—exception that has led to a surprising twist on the encounter between the King and the bathing woman. According to Phillipe Buc (1993):

> For many late twelfth- and thirteenth-century masters in the French schools, ... Bath-sheba was having her period (hence washing herself). Her menstrual flow stopped when she had intercourse with David: immediately at the touch of the king, because of the sanctity of the anointing.... it was widely believed that this anointing endowed the French kings with a miraculous power, the healing touch. (p. 102)

This view of the scripture is based on the Latin Vulgate version of the text, "*statimque sanctificata est ab immunditia sua*," which Buc translates into English as "She was instantly sanctified of her pollution" (p. 102). Buc builds his analysis on the fact that during the reign of the Capetian Kings in France (987–1328) the royalty chose for their role model the illustrious King David of Biblical fame. And one of the traits attributed to David, and which, therefore, they claimed as their own, was the power to heal, though it was mainly applied to healing scrofula.

Despite the desire to build up the powers of the rulers, nonetheless, it was a huge intellectual and cultural leap for them to have set aside, even for their kings, the social prohibitions against male contact with menstrual fluid as well as the biological understanding that menstrual sex was less likely to lead to pregnancy. Of course, once one enters the realm of miracles, anything is conceivable, but the story captures how far men have gone to cope with the mysterious "otherness" of a menstruating woman.

Unfortunately, there do not appear to be any documents that address whether or not King David's putative indifference to the notion of menstrual pollution due to carnal contact with menstrual blood led to a wider erosion of the taboo or made engagement in the act appealing. One can imagine the thought process: After all, if it was OK with King David and also resulted in the cessation of Bathsheba's flow, then it must be good for both the man and the woman. There is a striking modern sequel to this line of thought: it is becoming common to recommend sexual activity to women as a way to relieve menstrual pain due to the fact that the contractions induced by orgasm can relieve cramps.

Although it did not become part of later Christian belief in England, a similar interpretation of what went on between David and Bathsheba appeared in the Wycliffe Bible, one of the earliest efforts to create an English language version of the scriptures. The Wycliffe translation emerged over a period of years (1382–1395) and it too attributed menstrual healing powers to the King:

> Then by messengers sent, David took her; and when she entered to him, he slept with her, and anon she was hallowed from her uncleanness. And she turned again into her house, with a child conceived; and she sent, and told to David, and said, I have conceived. (2 Samuel 11:2–5)

Years later, during the 15th century C.E., a golden age of the illuminated manuscript, the moment of David's spying upon Bathsheba as she cleansed herself following the end of her period became a popular subject for the artists who prepared the finely rendered page paintings that were bound within the covers of the books that were prepared for the wealthy merchants and nobility as well as for high ranking clergy. The pictures are remarkably voluptuous and suggestive. The horny older man peers down upon the unsuspecting woman who is almost always shown from the front with breasts bared, sometimes cupping one of her breasts or touching herself. And to make the scene even more erotic, there is commonly a long thin object in the scene, often a fountain that is spurting water from its tip. Other symbolically apt details frequently appear. And in order to assure the viewer that Bathsheba is not menstruating, some of the images include objects such as a discarded red robe, pieces of red fruit or even red slippers laid to the side, a sign of her cast off earthiness.

Across the ages for theologians and others conducting exegetical examinations of this scene (until recently all men, of course) the most enduring debate regarding Bathsheba's behavior in the bathing scene has been whether she was an innocent target of King David's lust (he was already known to have had multiple sexual partners) or if she was a temptress who flaunted her body in order to seduce the King. Some have even claimed that the reference to her having been "cleansed" meant that she knew she was at the fertile point in her cycle and most likely to conceive. (It seems that the notion that women use pregnancy to entrap men into marriage is an ancient one.)

Monica Ann Walker-Vadillo (2008) has thoroughly explored these competing tropes in an insightful monograph whose subtitle captures the quandary: *Bathsheba in Late Medieval French Manuscript Illuminations: Innocent Object of Desire or Agent of Sin?* The book claims that, "The visual representation of David spying Bathsheba in her bath and of his sexual intercourse with her was a very popular topic in medieval art, in particular in the fifteenth and sixteenth century" (p. ii). However, this observation could easily be extended across a much broader historical spectrum. The more interesting point Vadillo makes is that distribution and consumption of the more explicit visual representations of the bathing scene were severely limited to particular, select audiences. The images were deemed inappropriate for some and readily available to others. In fact, for the elite owners of explicit manuscripts,

> It was believed that certain types of lascivious images should be placed in the bedchamber where they would arouse desire in the married couple while at the same time giving them an image of beauty to gaze upon so that the children that they conceived would possess beauty, health, and charm. (p. 78)

The point I wish to emphasize here is that these images, and the encounter being depicted, are of a post-menstrual, or non-menstrual encounter. It is crucial to the plot line (the resulting pregnancy) as well as to the aesthetic, social, psychological, and theological sensibilities of the entire community that there be no chance of menstrual taint. I contend that such values had become so thoroughly ingrained as to be non-conscious operational presumptions. And, to go a step further, for the most part, the same set of values and presumptions continue to operate today.

In contrast to the two tales of older men, Laban and David, and their troubled encounters with menstruating women, a New Testament story puts a very different, surprising spin on a menstrual transaction.

The story of Jesus as menstrual hero is found in Matthew 9: 18–26; Mark 5:21–43; and Luke 8:42–48. It occurred at a moment in his career when Jesus had become an established miracle worker, attracting throngs of supplicants wherever he went, constantly surrounded by a coterie of disciples. One day as Jesus was entering a town, he was beset by crowds beseeching him to perform healing miracles, including a request by a leader of the temple, a man named Ja'irus, who begged Jesus to save his dying daughter. In the crowd was a woman who, as the scriptures tell it, "had a flow of blood for twelve years and could not be healed by anyone" (Luke, 8:43). We can't be sure of the cause of her malady, but today she might be diagnosed as suffering from menorrhagia, heavy, irregular menstrual bleeding, or Von Willebrand Disease, a rare blood clotting disorder (today she might be prescribed a drug like Depo-Provera to regulate her menstrual cycle). To the people of her time she'd be little more than a leper, shunned by all, especially by the men of the community who were observant of the strictures spelled out in

Leviticus. The woman knew how she should behave, but her plight drove her to attempt a desperate act: having heard of the wondrous healing powers of this new messiah, she furtively slipped through the crowd, crawled up behind Jesus, and touched the hem of this robe. Jesus sensed the contact and said, "Who was it that touched me?" (Luke, 8:45).

Peter and the other disciples who saw the woman immediately panicked; they knew full well that if the woman had made contact, Jesus was soiled, and, as the menstrual dominos fell, they too were at risk if they had contact with him. Much was at stake, so everyone pretended nothing had happened: "When all denied it, Peter said, 'Master, the multitudes surround you and press upon you!'" (Luke, 8:45). But Jesus would have none of this lie, and then he did an amazing thing. He blatantly defied the menstrual rules of order by treating her as though the ancient taboo was a matter of no consequence. His statement to her became a staple of future faith-healing practices, "Daughter, your faith has made you whole; go in peace" (Luke, 8:48). Her menorrhagia was cured and he then went on to heal the daughter of Ja'irus (New King James Version).

As remarkable as this story is in the context of its own time and place, the fact that the menstrual detail in the story has gotten so little attention in the ensuing centuries strikes me as even more noteworthy. The fact that its implications are so discomforting may explain why it has seldom been depicted in classical paintings, illuminated manuscripts or other image media. Though the story has become one of the miracle tales, the part having to do with a man's defiance of the menstrual taboo is unsung. Jesus' rejection of other social norms is commonly praised, and sometimes emulated, but the power of the menstrual laws has trumped even Christ's pointed flaunting of them, with one significant exception: the story of Pope Gregory and St. Augustine of Canterbury.

It is interesting to try to determine why any particular cultural practice takes root in one place but not in another, even under the same religious umbrella or cultural context. Why did some groups embrace circumcision and others give it scant regard? Why kneeling in prayer for some and not for others? Why head coverings for one and none for others? And, why do some sub-groups or sects within a single faith hold fast to restricting women's participation in ritual events and avoid sexual relations during the period while others make little or no mention of it?

Two early Christian theologians, both who came to be known as Saint Augustine, made mention of menstruation. One was Augustine of Hippo (354–430), author of several highly regarded treatises, including *Confessions, The Literal Meaning of Genesis, The City of God* and other influential texts. The other was Augustine of Canterbury (died 604). The former spent years striving to reconcile carnality with procreation, carnality being the basis of original sin and man's expulsion from the Garden of Eden while sexual congress was a necessity for the perpetuation of the species. He identified the menstrual cycle as a sign of the original purity of humans, existing prior to Eve's giving in to the Devil's temptation because, a "… menstrual flux can now be produced from the womb of a virgin without loss of maidenhood" (Greenblatt, 2017, p. 28). The Augustine who rose to prominence several centuries later was focused on a more practical question.

Other than its commitment to the continuance of the "no menstrual sex" edict of ancient scriptures, there is little additional reference in the evolution of Christianity to menstrual restrictions, especially in Britain where there seem to be fewer folk lore taboos than exist in Italy and many Eastern European settings. This may be credited to Pope Gregory and his missionary to the heathen people of Britain, St. Augustine, who was declared the first Archbishop of Canterbury in 597. According to the history compiled by The Venerable Bede in the 8th century CE, Augustine wrote to the Pope asking for guidance on a number of topics, including the question of whether a menstruating woman could attend church. As he wrote in his letter, "These uncouth English people require guidance on all these matters" (p. 82).

Specifically citing the story of Christ and the bleeding woman, Pope Gregory responded this way:

> … a woman should not be forbidden to enter church during these times: for the workings of nature cannot be considered culpable, and it is not just that she should be refused admittance, since her condition is beyond her control. We know that the woman who suffered an issue of blood, humbly approaching behind our Lord, touched the hem of his robe and was at once healed of her sickness. If, therefore, this woman was right to touch our Lord's robe, why may not one who suffers nature's courses be permitted to enter the church of God? … So, if it was a laudable presumption in the woman who in her disease touched our Lord's robe, why may not the same concession be granted to all women who endure the weakness of their nature? A woman, therefore should not be forbidden to receive the mystery of Communion at these times. (p. 82)

A possible result was that the Old Testament rules of Leviticus received little attention and, therefore, did not get incorporated into the day-to-day sexual relationships of men and women in the new Christian lands, which were unfamiliar with ancient Abrahamic customs.

There are two long, continuous lines from Laban and Jesus to the present. The contrary ways that they responded to menstruating women have been played out with infinite variety across time and cultural variation. Laban's fear and disgust vs.

Jesus' indifference or even acceptance—these are the polar ends of the spectrum of male reactions to menstrual encounters. Between the poles of these transactions lie the nuanced stories that men have to tell. The stories are sometimes so subtle as to be barely remembered, while at other times they are deeply formative.

One of the most significant ways that Christianity differs from the two other faiths that emerged from the same geographic region and with which it shares some fundamental documents: the essential role that blood plays in the symbolism and belief system of the religion. Though Jewish and Islam studies make note of some of the blood sacrifices depicted in ancient texts, they do not place references to the shedding of blood, either symbolic or literal blood letting, at the core of the system. However, when viewed through the lens of menstrual conceptions, the story of Christ can be seen as a reenactment of the menstrual cycle. Christ performed the mysterious achievement that women do every month: he was able to bleed and not die. Or, to put it another way, he bled and after several days passed was resurrected.

Christianity has placed blood at the core of its system, including the concept of transubstantiation expressed through the ritual of communion and even in its architectural practices. Church doors are commonly painted blood red as it is "through the blood of Christ" that one enters the kingdom of heaven. As a boy growing up in a fundamentalist Baptist church in semi-rural Pennsylvania, I, and my church-mates, were regularly regaled with the story of Christ's bleeding on the cross and that the bleeding was Christ's gift to wash away man's sins. We were often encouraged to "accept the blood of Christ" and one of the hymns I can still hear ringing in my ears is one whose chorus goes, "There is power, power, wonder-working poser, in the blood of the Lamb" (Jones, 1899). Though Christianity is a patriarchal system, the men who wrote those songs and shaped the practices and beliefs were appropriating the menstrual rite of passage. "Washed in the blood" is one of the essential images of Protestantism, and it is through the symbolic enactment of this female biological phenomenon that one is "born again," just as it is through the shedding of the uterine lining that women themselves are readied to create new life.

Admittedly, this last speculative foray is a departure from the conventional historical explorations. It is not likely to be met with easy agreement—or any agreement at all. Let it serve as an example of how the richness of cultural constructions of the menstrual cycle can yield a never-ending range of speculation.

The ancient stories noted here, though few in number, vividly capture many of the perplexing nuances of menstrual transactions.

Note

For access to the images mentioned in this chapters, readers are directed to the Google Images data base and similar resources under headings such as "Laban Searching the Tents," "Bathsheba in the Bath," and "Jesus and the Bleeding Woman."

References

Bede. (1991). *Ecclesiastical history of the English people*. New York, NY: Penguin Classics.

Brozyna, M. (Ed.). (2005). *Gender and sexuality in the middle ages: A medieval source documents reader*. Jefferson, NC: McFarland

Buc, P. (1993). David's adultery with Bathsheba and the healing of Capetian Kings. *Viator, 24*, 101–120.

Diamant, A. (1997). *The Red Tent*. New York, NY: Picador.

Greenblatt, S. (2017, June 9). The invention of sex: St. Augustine's carnal knowledge. *The New Yorker, 93*(17), 24–28.

Jones, L. (1899). There is power in the blood. *Timeless Truths*. Retrieved July 3, 2017 from http://library.timelesstruths.org/music/There_Is_Power_in_the_Blood/

Plaut, G. (Ed.). (1981). *The Torah: A modern commentary*. New York, NY: Union of American Hebrew Congregations.

Sarna, N. (1966). *Understanding genesis*. New York, NY: Schocken Books.

Shlain, L. (2003). *Sex, time and power: How women's sexuality shaped human evolution*. New York, NY: Viking Press.

Updike, J. (2000). *Gertrude and Claudius*. New York, NY: Alfred A. Knopf.

Walker-Vadillo, M. (2008). *Bathsheba in late medieval French manuscript illumination: Innocent object of desire or agent of sin?* Lampeter: The Edwin Mellen Press.

Weltchronik. (1360). *Laban searching the tents*. Retrieved July 3, 2017 from Weltchronik, MS M.769 fol. 57r

CHAPTER THREE

A Royal Menstrual Pain

Prince Charles and the Tampon Scandal

"Oh, that I were a glove upon that hand that I might touch that cheek!"

Romeo, *Romeo and Juliet*, II, 1, 66–67
William Shakespeare

Mention the names "Prince Charles" and "Camilla Parker-Bowles" or more spe-cifically, "Camillagate" or "the Prince Charles tampon scandal," and those who remember anything about this 1993 piece of gossip will surely say something like, "Oh yeah, that's the story about the Prince of Wales wanting to be a tampon." Thus the words "tampon" and "Prince Charles" have become inextricably linked in popular imagination and memory. In fact, if you list those two terms in a Google search, you will be told that there are well over 600,000 items to look at, though many are zany or weird personal web sites that actually have little to do with the scandal. Similarly, a Lexis/Nexis search will yield more than 200 hits, depending on whether you use the term "tampon" or "Tampax."

Coverage of this story in the popular media went through twists and turns that offer a glimpse into one couple's intimate fantasies regarding the menstrual transaction as well as a full frontal view of the larger society's public attitudes and assumptions about appropriate behavior when it comes to the topic of menstru-ation. It also illustrates how deeply conflicted menstrual values are and how the topic can be appropriated as a rhetorical weapon in social and political discourse. But before delving into the layered meanings of the story, it is necessary to review the details of the event itself.

Even before the marriage of Charles, the Prince of Wales and heir to the British throne, to Diana Spencer, a relatively unknown 19-year-old, the British press, and to a lesser extent the celebrity reporting press of the rest of the former British colonies, including the U.S., devoured the tid bits of the couple's private life with an avidity matched only by the attention given the Kennedy family's travails in the United States. I wrote, "even before the marriage" because the first sexually titillating news item concerning the couple came with the announcement that before the marriage plans could be completed, Diana had to undergo a gynecological exam, conducted in order to assure the royal family that she was indeed a virgin. This in turn led to speculation about the possible effects of tampon use on the reliability of the intact hymen as an indicator of sexual innocence. The bride-to-be reassured the public, not to mention her fiancé and the Queen, that she was in fact chaste by saying, "I knew I had to keep myself tidy for what lay ahead" (Arndt, 2002, p. 1). This quaint phrasing evokes provocative associations to aspects of feminine hygiene that would come to haunt her husband more than a decade later.

From time to time rumors surfaced that either Charles or Diana was involved in extramarital sexual relations. While the men thought to be involved with Diana changed over time, one woman's name repeatedly came up in association with Charles: Camilla Parker-Bowles, a married woman and mother of two children.

The lives of all three individuals and perhaps even the nature of celebrity reporting and the status of British royalty, were radically altered in 1993. The impact of the story on all those involved, both at the most personal level and on a global media level, is testimony to the remarkable symbolic power menstruation has as a token of meaning.

Beginning with a story in an Australian women's magazine, *New Idea*, on January 13, 1993, a date that the Royals quickly came to refer to as "Black Wednesday," though "Red Wednesday" or "Bloody Wednesday" would have been more apt given the nature of the story, tabloids, followed by broadcast media and eventually more moderate media outlets, reported summaries and some excerpts of a mobile phone conversation that had actually taken place more than three years earlier on December 18, 1989. The gist of the story, echoed repeatedly around the world, was that Charles told Camilla that he fantasized about being reincarnated as a tampon so he could live inside her.

There are at least two especially interesting things about this reporting. First, in spite of the fact that anything relating to menstruation, at least in 1993, was broadly seen as an unmentionable topic in "polite" company and certainly one which was never discussed in association with sexual practices, here it was being extensively covered in even the more established outlets. The second, perhaps even more remarkable, detail is that virtually all of the reports got the story wrong, misreporting or misrepresenting the actual exchange between the lovers and completely reversing Charles's actual feelings and fantasies. I believe it is fair to say that whenever facts are sharply skewed or altered, it is probable that some vital social norms are being either challenged or protected or that lies are being told to promote the interests of those disseminating the lies.

In order to provide an accurate account of the exchange that shocked and outraged press and public alike, the pertinent passages are reprinted below. At this point in their lives Charles and Camilla had been lovers for years but often found it difficult to be together privately. On the night of the fateful phone call they were apparently feeling lonely and in need of one another both emotionally and sexually. In the midst of a series of passionate, explicit sexual remarks, the following exchange occurs:

Charles:	Oh God. I'll just live inside your trousers or something. It would be much easier!
Camilla:	(Laughing) What are you going to turn into, a pair of knickers? (both laugh) Oh, you're going to come back as a pair of knickers.
Charles:	Or God forbid a Tampax. Just my luck! (Laughs)
Camilla:	You are a complete idiot! (Laughs) Oh, what a wonderful idea.
Charles:	My luck to be chucked down the lavatory and go on and on forever swirling round on the top, never going down!
Camilla:	(Laughing) Oh, Darling!
Charles:	Until the next one comes through.
Camilla:	Or perhaps you could come back as a box.
Charles:	What sort of box?
Camilla:	A box of Tampax, so you could just keep going.
Charles:	That's true.
Camilla:	Repeating yourself … (Laughing) Oh, darling I just want you now. (Graham, 2001, p. 178)

The conversation goes on for another four minutes or so of banter, gossip and more longing before they ring off.

Let us focus on the precise way the two references to Tampax, a specific brand name that gets lost in most of the ensuing reportage, are used. First, when Charles says that he wants to live in Camilla's trousers, he hasn't identified himself as anything other than himself, presumable a tiny, sort of Lilliputian prince. Camilla introduces the idea of transformation to some other form, "a pair of knickers," or as Americans would say, a pair of panties. Charles, feeling glum and frustrated, responds, "Or, God forbid, a Tampax. Just my luck!" He makes the picture even bleaker by seeing himself not as a fresh tampon entering her vagina but as a discarded Tampax, "chucked down the lavatory ... forever swirling round the top, never going down." Camilla demonstrates her loving kindness by trying to put a positive spin on this pathetic self-pity by saying, "... perhaps you could come back as a box, ... a box of Tampax, so you could just keep going." Camilla sees the metaphoric possibilities in the tampon as something that is always ready and able to be put to use thereby countering Charles' view of its— and his—disposability.

Now consider the way the story was reported. Here's a representative sample of excerpts from articles that appeared in the weeks following the transcript's appearance in the Australian women's magazine:

The Ottawa Citizen (1993, January 14) reported that the transcripts, "aroused intense debate Wednesday over whether he would ever become king. ... Charles jokes that he wishes he could be turned into a Tampax..." (p. A-1).

MacLean's (1993) magazine said, "The awful ... tapes indeed had Charles wishing he might be a ladies' sanitary device in the next world ... I couldn't ever take a monarch who thinks like that seriously. Why didn't he quote one of our great poets, Pope or Dryden perhaps, and come back as his beloved's handkerchief or flea?" (p. 13).

Newsweek (1993) reported, "In a phone call with Camilla Parker-Bowles, Prince Charles fantasized about living 'inside your trousers' and being reborn as her tampon" (p. 8).

In *The Houston Chronicle* (1993, January 14) we read, "At another spot Charles jokes that he wishes he could be turned into a tampon" (p. 16).

The London *Sunday Times* (1993) said the transcript reads, "Like a limp schoolboy attempt at erotica" (n.p.). (What they mean to imply by the phrase "limp schoolboy" is both puzzling and suggestive.)

And in the *South China Morning Post* (1993) we read, "In the tape the prince is claimed to wish he could be reincarnated as one of Mrs. Parker-Bowles' tampons" (p. 1).

Even one year later *The Toronto Star* (1994) asked its readers, "Did you know that the Italian press has christened Charles 'Il tampolina'? That means the little tampon" (p. D-10).

It was also claimed that young women in America and Britain were going to pharmacies asking for a "box of Charlies" (Graham, 2001, p. 72).

As a media phenomenon, this is not a story that hit for a brief while and then quickly faded. As they say in the business, "This story had legs." Reporters and columnists had no qualms about passing judgments on Charles' alleged fantasies but went even further to offer opinions about what his fantasies suggested about his fitness to ascend to the throne. He's been called "smutty and juvenile" in *The Washington Post* (Cohen, 1998, p. W20), that he "can't seriously be a king after that" in the South African *Financial Mail* (Wilhelm, 1994, p. 1). *The Guardian* (Hoggart, 1998, p. 17) in London asked, "Can this man ever be king?" In Hong Kong the *South China Morning Post* (Walen, 1993, p. 1) reported the "British monarchy was thrown into even deeper crisis." *U.S.A. Today* (Williams, 1993, p. 12) suggested, "If that's his idea of romance, he should stick to chats with his plants." The New York *Daily News* (Tamposky, 1995, p. 5) added, "The prince apparently was so overwhelmed by his passion that two years ago he told [Camilla] he wished to be reincarnated as her tampon."

Even the rare article that expressed sympathy for the Prince still got the details of the story wrong, using it, as in the following case, as an excuse to take a swipe at some traditional religious practices and demonstrate the (male) writer's own sexual liberation:

> As it happens, the only time I've ever felt any affection for Prince Charles was when he told his beloved Camilla Parker-Bowles that he'd like to be one of her tampons. Apart from being raunchy, earthy and passionate, it suggested Charles doesn't share the ancient horrors of menstruation in many a major religion that denies women admission to church or temple when they're "unclean." (Adams, 1997, p. R02)

One could go on at greater length with newspaper and magazine citations, but the story doesn't stop with print media coverage. For instance, one month after the scandal broke, *Adweek* ("Camillagate faux pas," 1993) magazine reported, "On Jan. 17, four days after publication of the piquant terms of a telephone conversation .... an [ad] agency based in Sao Paulo—published a newspaper ad for Tampax, with the headline 'Approved even by the prince'" (n.p.).

There's more: In 1994 a play opened off Broadway called *Loose Lips* consisting in part of an enactment of the transcript. One review stated, "The biggest laugh comes as Camilla lustily suggests he 'could come back as a box ... a box of Tampax so you could just keep going.'" The review goes on to quote the director as claiming that his goal was not to make fun of the hapless couple but to make a point about intrusive media, "The play is a warning to people to think before they open their mouths because everyone's privacy is so easily pirated these days" (Gardiner, 1994, p. 5).

It wasn't long before American television got into the act with a sketch featuring Dana Carvey and Luke Perry on *Saturday Night Live* that replicated the famous announcement of King Edward VIII renouncing his throne "for the woman I love." In this case, however, the Prince Charles character explained that he was doing so in order to have himself turned into a tampon. The sketch uses actual footage from the December 10, 1936 newsreels of the time showing British families gathered around their radios listening to the abdication statement. Then it proceeds to a laboratory scene like those in science fiction films in which transformations take place, and we see the Prince changed into a tampon with his tiny head on top. Finally, he is delivered to the Parker-Bowles estate and handed to his lover in a gift-wrapped Tampax box by a mincing butler played by Mick Jagger. Camilla, however, has reconciled with her husband and tosses the tampon prince to the floor where he is discovered by a sniffing poodle dog.

Even the famously careful *New Yorker* (Amis, 2002) magazine got the story wrong in a review of a *Diana* biography with this catty remark: "So we come to 1992, ... that November it was revealed that Charles had been recorded while having a[n] ... intimate chat with Camilla Parker-Bowles. Long intrigued by the idea of the transmigration of souls, Charles saw himself reborn as, 'God forbid, a Tampax,' so that he could 'just live inside your trousers'" (p. 106).

What are we to make of this? Among the possible explanation, consider the following.

First, we have a glimpse into the dark recesses of Western culture's misogynistic views as expressed via references to one of the unique features of women's biology, their menstrual cycle. Ironically, Charles himself felt that to be cast in the role of an object performing a common feminine hygiene service was something that God should forbid, yet to even mention menstruation in the context of erotic relations was seen by the media establishment, which, at least in this case probably accurately reflects more widely held views, as so repugnant as to warrant distortion and the employment of those most powerful instruments of social control and discipline: ridicule and disgust.

In Euro-American culture it seems that the worst wish a little boy could make, the most unacceptable fantasy ambition he could express, would be, "When I grow up I want to be a woman." (This dynamic is dramatized touchingly in the film *Ma Vie en Rose*, 1997.) Tampons are so thoroughly "gendered" items, and so thoroughly beyond the pale of the male domain, that they represent some sort of essence of woman that men may have no truck with. It is a commonplace that many men feel discomfort and embarrassment even shopping for menstrual products let alone having physical contact with them in use, and, by implication, with the bodily fluid they are meant to absorb, menstrual blood.

Mary Jane Lupton (1993) and others have effectively demonstrated the pervasiveness of the menstrual taboo which may even out rank homosexuality as "the sin that dare not speak its name." Lupton's study of the menstrual gap in Freud's work and in psychoanalysis in general emphasizes the idea that, avoidance … reflects larger cultural attitudes, not only toward menstruation but toward female sexuality. Because menstruation has been consistently silenced by institutions such as the family, the educational system, and the church, it is apt to be silenced in a theoretical work—called by another name or otherwise disguised. (Lupton, 1993, p 3)

By even entertaining the thought of becoming a tampon, Charles has crossed a line, he has "gone over to the other side." In effect, he has become that most vile of creatures, a traitor to his kind, in this case, a gender traitor. And for this transgression he receives the same punishment that betrayers commonly encounter: he is shunned, banished, publicly denounced as severely as Hawthorne's Hester Prynn was, made to wear the bloody tampon around his neck. It remains to be seen if, when his mother dies, he will be able to ascend the throne without yet another review of this (to use appropriate British vernacular) bloody awful story.

Second, the story suggests deep feelings of ambivalence about class structure and its gender aspects. On one hand, the reports took glee in this opportunity to pull the Prince off the throne by associating him with a woman's private product. The magazine *New Statesman* (Riddell, 1996) even ran a headline calling him "an amorous Tampax" (p. 1). Yet at the same time the ire and ridicule seemed to suggest a conservative longing for the kind of royalty that always behaved well and provided sterling role models everyone could look up to. Or, as *The Guardian* (Hoggart, 1995) of London put it, condemning both Charles and Diana, "After last night will anyone in a dinner jacket lift a glass and say, 'gentlemen, the King?' Would Americans salute a flag with 13 tampons in the top left corner? Let us hope they sort it out and disappear gracefully before the Queen dies" (p. 17).

The idea of Americans saluting a British flag, with or without tampons, is an expression of nostalgia on a par with those Confederate flags that still wave over some sad Southern outposts. Or, perhaps the writer meant to say that the Brits were wimps for putting up with such unmanly doings because, after all, Americans (real men!) would never tolerate it. And that's probably right. President Clinton was forgiven (if approval ratings mean anything) for his crass cigar sex play with Ms. Lewinsky but surely would have been booted out if instead he savored her tampon with the same gusto.

However, in spite of the drubbing that Charles took, it is conceivable that the "outing" of his and Camilla's tampon eroticism was a contributing factor in what has become a steady increase in the acceptability of menstrual references in public media including TV drama and sit-com references to menarche, PMS and menopause as well as satires and jokes on comedy programs. Just as Clinton's escapades made oral sex a common topic, so did those of Prince Charles move menstruation at least part way out of the closet.

Third, the story suggests that when it comes to menstruation and sex, the two don't mix. Of course, this is simply a reflection of strongly held Judeo-Christian beliefs. In fact, apparently Charles's relationship with his wife, Princess Diana, was governed by those values as well for it has been reported that when Diana heard the story she told her private secretary, "God, Patrick, a Tampax! That's sick" ("Work-and-tell," 2000, September 25, p. 10).

The nearly universal expressions of displeasure at what came to be the accepted story of the sexual fantasies of Charles and Camilla reveal a set of social values that Jonathan Dollimore has explored in *Sex, Literature and Censorship*. Though Dollimore concentrated on the "disgust" often expressed towards homoerotic practices, his analysis is apt: "Disgust is typically experienced at the boundaries of a culture, and of the individual identities of those who belong to it, and its focus is typically what is excluded by those boundaries and especially what is just the other side of them" (p. 47). What is "just the other side" of Charles's identity in this case is the feminine. As this story indicates, one crosses that boundary at one's peril.

Finally, consider another of the many peculiar ironies in this menstrual tale. Earlier I noted a line from *MacLean's* (Amiel, 1993) magazine lamenting that Charles had not quoted a great poet such as Pope or Dryden who wanted to "come back as his beloved's handkerchief or flea." A review of English literature suggests that even this detail is wrong. It was neither Pope nor Dryden who wrote about a lover identifying with a flea, but John Donne who, early in the 17th century, wrote a delightfully raunchy poem titled "The Flea" that might be taken to be implying oral sex. The conceit has the speaker asking the woman he lusts after why he can't have the same privilege as a flea that has bitten her. As he puts it,

> It sucked me first, and now sucks thee,
> And in this flea our two bloods mingled be;
> Thou know'st that this cannot be said
> A sin, nor shame, nor loss of maidenhead,

The poem mentions mingling blood three times as well as other suggestive imagery. Why the *MacLean's* columnist finds this sort of poetic license attractive while condemning the Prince and Camilla for their tampon reference tells us more about today's sexual values than it does about poetry. A more fitting literary allusion might have been to the Shakespearean lines that begin this chapter. Romeo Prince Charles and his Juliet Camilla have simply updated the medium through which their longing is expressed.

Note

This chapter was previously published as "Camillagate: Prince Charles and the Tampon Scandal" in *Sex Roles: A Journal of Research*. (2006, March). Vol. 54, (5–6), 347–351. Reprinted by permission from Springer Nature.

References

Adams, P. (1997, March 29). Keep an eye on the watchdog. *The Weekend Australian*, p. R02. Retrieved May 18, 2002, from Lexis-Nexis Academic Universe database.

Amiel, B. (1993, February 1). Charles, Diana and the role of the media. *MacLean's*, p. 13. Retrieved May 18, 2003, from Lexis-Nexis Academic Universe database.

Amis, M. (2002, May 20). The queen's heart. *The New Yorker*, p. 106. Retrieved May 18, 2003, from Lexis-Nexis Academic Universe database.

Arndt, B. (2002, September 21). Whatever happened to virginity? *The Age*, p. 1. Retrieved May 18, 2003, from Lexis-Nexis Academic Universe database.

Camillagate faux pas in Brazil. (1993, February 22). *Adweek*, np. Retrieved May 18, 2003, from Lexis-Nexis Academic Universe database.

Cohen, R. (1998, February 22). Wired eyes: How tapes and technology freeze our times–and sometimes the blood itself. *The Washington Post*, p. w20. Retrieved May 18, 2003, from Lexis-Nexis Academic Universe database.

Dollimore, J. (2001). *Sex, literature and Censorship*. Cambridge, UK: Polity Press.

Donne, J. (1633) *The flea*. Retrieved July 3, 1917 from https://www.poetryfoundation.org/poems/46467/the-flea

Gardiner, D. (1994, August 14). Camilla tape is talk of the town. *The People*, p. 5. Retrieved May 18, 2003, from Lexis-Nexis Academic Universe database.

Gould, S. (1981). *Mismeasure of man*. New York, NY: W.W. Norton.

Graham, C. (2001). *Camilla: Her true story*. London: John Blake Publishing. Hoggart, S. (1995, November 21). The Di is cast. *The Guardian*, p. 17. Retrieved April 12, 2003, from Lexis-Nexis Academic Universe database.

Howard, L., & Cerio, G. (1993, November 8). Knickers snickers. *Newsweek*, p. 8. Retrieved May 18, 2003, from Lexis-Nexis Academic Universe database.

Lupton, M. (1993). *Menstruation and psychoanalysis*. Chicago, IL: Unveristy of Illinois Press.

No 900 number necessary. (1993, January 14). *The Houston Chronicle*, p. 16. Retrieved September 10, 2002, from Lexis-Nexis Academic Universe database.

Riddell, M. (1996, July 5). He's been a whinging son, a sulking husband and, in his dream, an amorous Tampax. *New Statesman*, p. 1. Retrieved October 10, 2002, from Lexis-Nexis Academic Universe database.

The royal soap opera. (1993, January 14). *The Ottawa citizen*, p. A1. Retrieved May 17, 2003, from Lexis-Nexis Academic Universe database.

Samson, P. (1993, January 17). Of thrones and phones. *Sunday Times*, np. Retrieved September 10, 2002, from Lexis-Nexis Academic Universe database.

Smyth, M. (1994, February 27). Diane still woos the limelight despite her lingering goodbye. *The Toronto Star*, p. D10. Retrieved April 12, 2003, from Lexis-Nexis Academic Universe database.

Tamposky, E. (1995, December 21). Queen sez di-vorce now. *Daily News*, p. 5. Retrieved April 12, 2003, from Lexis-Nexis Academic Universe database.

Tavris, C. (1992). *The mismeasure of woman*. New York, NY: Simon & Schuster.

Walen, D. (1993, January 14). Charles details sex fantasies in phone chat with Camilla. *South China Morning Post*, p. 1. Retrieved May 17, 2003, from Lexis-Nexis Academic Universe database.

Wilhelm, P. (1999, February 12). Only the goldfish is pure. *Financial Mail*, p. 4. Retrieved May 18, 2003, from Lexis-Nexis Academic Universe database.

Williams, J. (1993, January 6). Julia Roberts' pretty words for movie exec. *U.S.A. Today*, p. 2D. Retrieved May 17, 2003, from Lexis-Nexis Academic Universe database.

Work-and-tell author still defiant. (2000, September 25). *The Herald*, p. 10. Retrieved May 17, 2003, from Lexis-Nexis Academic Universe database.

The world on Charles at 50. (1998, November 21). *The Guardian*, p. 5. Retrieved May 17, 2003, from Lexis-Nexis Academic Universe database.

CHAPTER FOUR

The Literary Period

Sightings, Sex, and Dystopian Visions

Perhaps the most significant single decade in the history of menstrual transactions appearing in published fiction was the 1970s. Beginning with Judy Blume's path breaking novel *Are You There God, It's Me, Margaret* (1970) and Toni Morrison's *The Bluest Eye* in the same year through Erika Jong's *Fear of Flying* (1973), Stephen King's *Carrie* (1974), Tom Robbins' *Even Cowgirls Get the Blues* (1976), and Scott Spencer's *Endless Love* (1979) writers recognized that menstruation played an important role in people's lives, and they included its presence in the stories they told. I have written an in depth look of the decade's literary menstrual cycle in a previously published chapter titled "The Decade Gets Its Period," and readers are directed to that source for the full discussion: *American Literature in Transition, 1970–1980*. Curnutt, K., (Ed.) (2018), New York: Cambridge University Press.

Due to the nature of publication practices it is not possible to create a comprehensive catalog of menstrual transactions in novels. Such moments are often fleeting and of little consequence. Furthermore, novels, unlike nonfiction, never come equipped with an index so that particular references can be easily identified. But in order to offer a sense of the variety of such incidents that do occur, the chapter concludes with a randomly gathered catalog of menstrual sightings. Though the list is admittedly idiosyncratic, it reflects the variety of menstrual transactions that novelists have noted and the many ways the topic affects relationships as well as its symbolic uses. Space restrictions do not allow for detailed annotation of the works so the reader is left to recall or discover the menstrual elements within.

But first, the chapter begins with an examination of two particular kinds of menstrual transactions that warrant special scrutiny. One involves what happens to fundamental social arrangements when the menstrual cycle goes awry or is radically altered, a situation I call "menstrual dystopia." The other has to do with the most private, intimate element in relationships: how couples manage sex in the presence of the period.

Dystopian Visions

Two of the most enduring tropes in literary fiction are the conceptions of the nearly perfect and, conversely, the generally imperfect, world, the utopian vs. dystopian vision. Customarily, dystopian stories depict societies in which nearly everyone has been reduced to a state of mindless obedience or tyrannical subjugation due to the rise of an overwhelming force that has taken control of the minds and daily lives of the people, such as in H. G. Wells' *The Time Machine* (1895), George Orwell's *1984* (1949), Aldus Huxley's *Brave New World* (1932) or *A Clockwork Orange* (1962) by Anthony Burgess. The work of Wells, Orwell, Huxley and most others focus on male characters and their struggles against the plight that has befallen the society and the way the spirit and independence of its citizens have been broken.

All such conjectures, whether in novels or intellectual explorations into social phenomena, constitute cautionary tales, efforts to grab the reader by the lapels and direct attention to a threat, a possibility, a fear of some dire consequence that is lurking just beyond our awareness.

Exceptions to the pattern set by male authors featuring male characters are found in two more recent novels, Margaret Atwood's *The Handmaid's Tale* (1985) and Ann Patchett's *State of Wonder* (2011). These two are unique because the main characters are women and because the plot centers on questions, in one case, about how a social/political/economic system might respond to a disruption in the reproductive lives of its female members or, in another, how individuals and the pharmaceutical industry might respond to the discovery of a means of extending women's reproductive capacity indefinitely.

The plots defy the "natural" order of the known (and presumably eternal) biological world. These are disturbing new worlds. In one, pregnancy is rare and the earth's human population is in danger of extinction. In the other world a different supernatural event is unfolding, a Garden of Eden in which a woman from the "civilized" world, Dr. Annick Swenson, a New Age Eve, can retreat to a remote paradise and have a baby at the age of 73. The story goes beyond Rousseau's refutation of the modern world to include a rejection of Darwinian evolution.

The titles of both works invite readers to view them in the tradition of folklore, fables or even mythology. *The Handmaid's Tale* is told in the first person but we learn at the end of the book that we have been reading a document transcribed from a trove of 30 audio cassettes that were discovered by scholars who are presenting their findings many years beyond the events being described at a conference hosted by the Department of Caucasian Anthropology at the University of Denay, Nunavit. (Why Atwood decided to use this silly pun as the name of a university escapes me; perhaps it is in keeping with the parody of academic papers that wraps up the narrative.)

Patchett employs a similarly fanciful device for the title of her book, *A State of Wonder*, suggesting a soft, fairy tale ambiance for a story full of dark undertones. Perhaps it would be more accurate to call Patchett's story an example of speculative fiction since it takes place in the present and imagines a remote tribal community, the Lakashi People, in which the consumption of a rare tree bark secretion has altered the menstrual cycle so that women do not experience menopause but continue to ovulate, become pregnant, and bear children no matter how old they are, despite the fact that the rest of their biological functions proceed through the same aging processes as women everywhere else.

Patchett is giving a twist to the mythic tale of Ponce de Leon's search for the fountain of youth. It is as though his quest has been fulfilled but with an ironic twist. Surely he sought an elixir that would grant *men* the vitality, strength, appearance and sexual vigor of their "prime." He would have been perplexed or indifferent to a substance that endowed women with extended childbearing capacity without the other traits associated with feminine youth. Patchett brings together the kind of "primitive" setting in which Ponce de Leon expected to find the source of eternal youth with "modern" scientific explorations such as those undertaken by drug companies that hope to reap enormous profit from the discovery of solutions to social, medical or biological "problems."

The novel addresses a new phenomenon in women's reproductive lives: the practice of delaying the age at which women have children. A not fully anticipated consequence of delaying one's plans to conceive until one's 30s or 40s is, for a variety of reasons, often a lowered likelihood of conception and carrying successfully to term, as well as a tendency to have fewer children. The rise of *in vitro* fertilization, surrogacy and adoption are some of the means of dealing with this development.

Building a plot around the discovery of a "cure" for age related infertility is an apt tale for our times. The dark side of the story involves an intersection between a small tribe of indigenous people located deep in the Amazon rain forests and the scientists who set up a research post in order to discover the source of their remarkable reproductive lives and create a way to reproduce the substance under industrial circumstances.

Like Joseph Conrad's Kurtz in *Heart of Darkness* (1899), the plot involves one of the researchers who "goes native," cutting ties with her drug company employers and settling into an ever-increasing alienation from her roots. But Patchett is not interested in the kind of power hungry, alienated male character that Conrad created. Rather than bringing back a vaccine against malaria, as her employers sent her to find, she has discovered a means of prolonging fertility. At one point she confides, "I will give them a drug that will, if anything, undermine the health of women and make them [the drug company] truly an obscene fortune" (pp. 288–289).

Her remark reveals a shrewd understanding that in capitalist economies a menstruating body is seen as a body in need of a consumer product. As she has done in other novels such as *The Patron Saint of Liars* (1992) and *Run* (2007) Patchett offer insightful perspectives on the lives and travails of modern women.

Since dystopian works are usually constructed with a "post-catastrophic" vision, one in which the imagined society is the result of some environmental or political disaster that has led to its depicted conditions, Patchett's book would not usually be categorized with other dystopian tales as it has a "primitive" setting in the present rather than a future culture; but it is full of implications about what would become of the social structure should the product become widely available. It might be thought of as "pre-catastrophic" in its vision. The predictions are dire and imagined rather than spelled. However, the ramifications of her story are as socially disruptive as those in other novels but in this case absent authoritarian forms of control mechanisms and power. A profound question about social arrangements lies at the heart of the investigation—and it all hinges on the ramifications of changes in the menstrual cycle.

In contrast, Margaret Atwood's *The Handmaid's Tale* and its successor adaptations for film and video serialization are constructed more within the dystopian tradition. Her focus on the impact of menstrual cycle disruption places women, both the Handmaids who are fertile and the wives of the Commanders who are not, at the center of the action.

While Patchett frames control of the menstrual cycle through the lens of consumer capitalism, the motivating factors in Atwood's fictional world are based on extreme religious and political conservatism. The decision makers in the fictional

Gilead are desperate to uphold traditional gender roles. The character through whom the story is told has been reduced to little more than a reproducing machine, the possessor of working ovaries and a healthy uterus. Everything in her life is constructed to reinforce that function. The most prominent physical reminder of her role is the use of the color red, a vivid display of a Handmaid's fecundity: she still has a menstrual cycle.

The Handmaids' shoes, gloves, shopping bags, bathrobes, the cloaks that cover their bodies, and even the cars used to transport them are red. "Everything except the wings around my face is red: the color of blood, which defines us" (p. 11). To further obliterate any sense of identity other than that of a reproductive system, the women are stripped of their names and referred to only by the name of the male Commander whose sperm they are required to accept in order to bear a child that will be given to the Commander's wife as though she had borne it. Thus, the narrator is known only as "Offred," and she understands that she is viewed as "a national resource" (p. 85). "We are two-legged wombs, that's all: sacred vessels, ambulatory chalices" (p. 176).

There is very little specific mention of menstruation itself, although every waking moment of the characters' lives is centered on whether or not a period will occur and the consequences of the outcome. The Handmaids themselves have internalized the collective worry: "Each month I watch for blood, fearfully, for when it comes it means failure. I have failed once again to fulfill the expectations of others, which have become my own" (p. 95). The fear is well founded. If too many months go by without a successful conception, the woman will be disgraced, declared unworthy of her special role and shipped off to a life of labor in the colonies or to some other menial role.

Given the rigid gender divisions within the society of Gilead, it is impermissible at any time to suggest that failure to conceive might be due to a problem with the Commander's reproductive apparatus. When a doctor who is giving Offred her monthly gynecological exam offers to make her pregnant himself and casually suggests that her Commander might be sterile, she responds in shock: "I almost gasp: he's said a forbidden word. *Sterile.* There is no such thing as a sterile man anymore, not officially. There are only women who are fruitful and women who are barren, that's the law" (p. 79). The centrality of the menstrual cycle's function has been so thoroughly codified so as to fully define women in its term but also to impose ever more rigid definitions on male identity as well. It turns out that the Commander's wife, who had been depicted as one of the architects of the Gilead theocracy has a cynical view of the system and suggests that perhaps Offred's failure to conceive is due to her husband's inadequacy. She offers to arrange for Offred to couple with some other man whose sperm might be more robust.

Offred's account ends ambiguously as she climbs into a van that will either take her to a safe haven to join the resistance or to punishment for "violation of state secrets," as one of the mysterious men who have come to fetch her explains to the Commander and his wife (p. 377). The lengthy coda that follows Offred's sudden departure is in the form of a parody of an academic conference. It is complete with smug observations by the presenting professors about being careful not to be overly judgmental and project their presumably more enlightened values upon the benighted citizens of the culture being examined.

Although somewhat heavy-handed, it is in this turn toward satire that Atwood broadens her field of vision. Her lecturing historian explains that they must take a detached view to the life and times of the Handmaids and their plight. The scholar does not mention menstruation specifically but does frame the history in the context of all of the conception management techniques that were in place at the time of the revolution that brought about the Gileadian Era. The techniques cited are familiar to readers of Atwood's book but are mere artifacts to those attending the academic conference in 2195.

There is an underlying warning within the coda. The social apocalypse that reduced women to little more than walking wombs had its roots in social history, which turns out to be contemporary America's social history. Atwood has given the dystopian tradition another dimension. Utilizing the allusions to contemporary reproductive techniques and technologies she has joined the ranks of Orwell and Huxley with her own version of the admonition, "Be careful what you wish for."

On the surface Atwood's story of the Handmaid and Ann Patchett's scientist plying her trade in the Amazon rain forest seem far removed from one another. But at the center of both is a dark concern with how the human reproductive system works and the management of the menstrual cycle itself.

Male Novelists Take on Menstrual Sex

Menstruation is a universal phenomenon in healthy women for more than 30 years of their lives, a fact that affects how men and women relate to one another in a myriad of ways, not least of which how they conduct their sexual relations. Yet, women in fiction seldom have periods. We might call this condition *literary amenorrhea*, the absence of menstrual cycles in fiction.

Despite the general avoidance of the subject, a few men have mentioned menstruation and a very few have even addressed it in the context of sexual encounters. Consider the work of three authors who have done so: Philip Roth, Scott Spencer,

and Bernard Malamud. Each writer has created scenes in which male characters become sexually involved with menstruating women. The way the scenes are
treated and how the characters themselves respond to the presence of menstrual
fluid reveal a variety of perspectives ranging from nearly fetishistic eroticization
to distaste and devastating consequences. And while each author has approached
the topic in a unique way, there are similar thematic and symbolic elements within
what we might call the menstrual trope.

In 1966 (the same year, incidentally, that feminine hygiene sprays were first
marketed) Bernard Malamud's novel *The Fixer* describes a character, Yakov Bok,
who wants nothing more than to live his life free of the entanglements of religious
and ethnic assumptions, yet he is constantly entrapped by the cultural baggage he
carries within and that is forced upon him from without. One piece of that baggage is the Jewish taboo against sex during menstruation. Yakov has been propo-
sitioned by Zina, the daughter of a bourgeoisie Russian businessman for whom he
has been working. She is an emotionally frail woman, headed for a life of spinster-
hood caring for her drunken father. Her wobbling gait, product of a deformed leg,
explains why she has remained single and also why the ever-sympathetic Yakov
agrees, against his better judgment, to have sex with her.

With fatally bad timing, Yakov enters her bedroom before she has finished
bathing and sees "a dribble of bright blood run down her crippled leg." He
exclaims, "But you are unclean!" Rather than seeing her period as an impedi-
ment to sex, Zina realizes its contraceptive advantage: "But surely you know this
is the safest time? ... And there's no inconvenience to speak of, the flow stops
the minute we begin." But Yakov recalls, "his wife's modesty during her period"
and replies, "Excuse me, some can, but I can't." Though he tries to leave politely,
Zina is hurt and angry. "'I'm a lonely woman, Yakov Ivanovitch,' she cried, 'have
mercy a little!'" (p. 46)

Yakov's rejection of Zina comes to haunt him when she accuses him of trying
to rape her and testifies against him in the magistrate's office. His situation is made
worse when he tells the investigators about Zina's period, embarrassing her and
making the court officers even more angry at his effrontery in revealing intimate
details about a frail, respectable Russian woman. Yet the Russians have their own
menstrual superstitions. When Yakiv tells the magistrate that he saw Zina's blood,
the Prosecuting Attorney comments sarcastically, "Did that have some religious
meaning for you as a Jew? Do you know that in the Middle Ages Jewish men
were said to menstruate?" (p. 82). Later, during his imprisonment, the authorities
become fixated on this notion:

[they] waited impatiently for his menstrual period to begin ... If it didn't start soon
they threatened to pump blood out of his penis with a machine they had for that

purpose. The machine was a pump made of iron with a red indicator to show how much blood was being drained out. The danger of it was that it didn't always work right and sometimes sucked every drop of blood out of the body. It was used exclusively on Jews; only their penises fitted it. (p. 123)

The juxtaposition of these two details—the authorities' posture of protecting the purity of Russian womanhood against contamination by contact with the feared and hated Jew, commonly expressed as "Jewish blood," and the attribution of menstruation to a male Jew—captures the vexed set of cultural values that menstruation is imbued with. Jewish men can be made to seem disgusting and emasculated if they can be so thoroughly feminized as to having periods. Although it seems that Russian Christian men are more comfortable with actual contact with menstrual blood during intercourse, the depth of their own misogyny is revealed in the belief that the hated Jewish male shares an essential characteristic of women.

Yet, an ironic note is revealed near the novel's end when we learn that the Tsar's son, Alexis, is a hemophiliac. In a fantasy conversation the Tsar tells Yakov, "Alexei's veins are fragile, brittle, and in the slightest mishap internal bleeding causes him unbearable pain and torment" (p. 303). The need to control blood and its symbolic meaning is reflected in both Jewish and Christian cultures. Yakov perpetuates his cultural heritage by avoiding menstrual blood during sex while the Russian Christians maintain their notion of their identity as Christians—or at least their non-Jewishness—by insisting that Jewish men menstruate. Malamud suggests that all the blood fetish is destructive to all parties as symbolized by the frailty of the Tsar's son who, beyond the fictional world of the novel, will soon come to bleed to death at the hands of the Bolshevik revolution.

In contrast, while Malmud's Yakov Bok avoids contact with menstrual blood, a decision that propels him toward his doom, some of Philip Roth's characters rush to embrace it, and one of them too is doomed in the process. Menstrual blood heightens sexual arousal for Roth's characters, both for its intimacy and for the erotic pleasure of violating the taboos against menstrual sex.

Roth has included sexual menstrual scenes in both *Sabbath's Theater* (1995) and *The Dying Animal* (2001). In the former, the sexually omnivorous Drenka describes the day she had sex with four different men and how during the third encounter she had a heavy menstrual flow. Following that coupling, the white towel the couple had placed under them is so spotted with blood and semen that the man cannot launder it at home for fear of his wife finding the evidence. Drenka blithely puts it in a plastic bag and takes it away with her. The inclusion of the menstrual sex scene serves the purpose of emphasizing how adventurous Drenka is, that she is constantly seeking new ways to explore both her own sexual capacities as well as those of the men she meets. But the even more thrilling erotic element for Drenka is in telling her lover Micky Sabbath about the experience. A characteristic of their illicit relationship is that they tell each other every intimate detail of their past and present sexual adventures. Both have extraordinary sexual histories and both seem completely devoid of any shame or jealousy. However, it may be noteworthy that Sabbath makes no mention of ever having engaged in menstrual sex himself, though for a man of his tastes and compulsions, it seems unlikely that he had any qualms in this department.

Six years and several novels later Roth returned to the subject with the publication of *The Dying Animal* in 2001. This time an ongoing Roth character, the scholar and professor, David Kepesh, another of Roth's womanizers, is brought to his knees—literally—by a menstruating woman.

Although Kepesh is a sexual predator who has seduced dozens of women, including many of his young students, he has become enraptured by Consuela Castillo, a recent graduate nearly 40 years his junior. Like Mickey Sabbath, he prides himself on his sexual prowess and on his ability to maintain emotional distance from his conquests, yet when Consuela tells him of a boyfriend who liked to witness her menstrual blood flow, he is shocked to realize that he has never done that himself and insists that she do the same for him. Though he doesn't say so, it appears as though he has had very little sexual contact with menstruating women. He is enthralled by the experience, but also overcome by her brazenness:

> ... when she shamelessly obliged, I wound up again intimidating myself. There seemed nothing to be done—if I wished not to be humbled completely by her exotic matter-of-factness—except to fall to my knees to lick her clean. Which she allowed to happen without comment. Making me into a still smaller boy. ... Each new excess weakening me further—yet what is an insatiable man to do? (pp. 71–72)

Kepesh's discovery of the erotic potential of menstrual blood embodies his awareness of life's limitations. He becomes irrationally jealous of the boy in his lover's past who was, as he describes it, "transfixed by the enigma of her discharge" (p. 46). His own fixation with Consuelo's, however, is linked to his growing awareness of his own mortality, as implied in the novel's title, *The Dying Animal*, which is an allusion to a line in a Yeats poem, "Sailing to Byzantium." Kepesh's only close male friend understands the psychological significance of his behavior and tells him:

> You violated the law of aesthetic distance. You sentimentalized the aesthetic experience with this girl... Do you know when that happened? The night she took the tampon out. The necessary aesthetic separation collapsed not while you watched her bleeding—that was all right, that was fine—but when you couldn't restrain yourself and went down on your knees... Worship me, she says, worship the mystery of the

bleeding goddess, and you do it. You stop at nothing. You lick it... She penetrates you... I'm not against it because it's unhygienic. I'm not against it because it's disgusting. I'm against it because it's falling in love. (p. 99)

Though Kepesh, like Micky Sabbath, has struggled to free himself of all cultural restraints and sentimentality, he finds himself mesmerized and emotionally enslaved by a young woman who will blithely share her menses with him. He who has prided himself on his power and control, particularly in the realm of sexual relationships, recapitulates the Biblical scene in the Garden of Eden when he ingests the streaming red fruit of her body and relinquishes his claims to sexual freedom and liberation—his own peculiar version of innocence—by falling in love.

While Malamud's Yakov Bok abides by the ancient menstrual taboo and suffers for his obedience, Roth's character defies the taboo and is punished as well; the former by social and political persecution and the latter by emotional torment. And in spite of the importance of the menstrual presence, neither Sabbath nor Kepesh actually engages in genital contact during a period. Scott Spencer's characters, however, revel in it.

Spencer's novel, *Endless Love* (1979), employs menstrual sex as a means of dramatizing an obsessive-compulsive love fixation that has run out of control. It is a modernized Romeo and Juliet story in which the young man in the tale accidentally burns down the home of his girl friend's family and later accidentally causes her father's death. Their graphically sexual encounter takes place in a hotel room while she is having a very heavy menstrual flow. By the time they have sated themselves with repeated couplings, the narrator tells us:

> We were both covered in dried blood. The sheets were stiff with it. If we hadn't put the chain on, the poor cleaning woman would have walked in on us and perhaps fainted. Immobile, we would have looked like the victims of a savage crime. There was blood on our legs, our thighs, our arms and fingers. There was blood in our hair and in the corners of our lips. Our lips themselves were caked with it. (p. 324)

These are the last sentences of a 26-page scene, most of which details the sexual encounter and the presence of Jade's blood. The portion of the passage describing them as looking like "victims of a savage crime" is symbolically apt. On the surface the description of menstrual sex in Spencer's novel is lusty and positive. It is clear that they have had menstrual sex before and are comfortable not only with the blood but with the menstrual paraphernalia as well. Jade casually tosses her pad over the edge of the bed and David sensuously twirls his finger around the string of her tampon to remove it. There is no discrete slipping off to the bathroom to attend to "private" matters for this randy couple. Rather than being restrained by the presence of Jade's period, they are erotically charged. Beneath the free flow of menstrual blood lies the history of their ill-fated affair and the dark future that awaits them. David is doomed to spend years incarcerated in a psychiatric prison and the rest of his life mourning the loss of his idealized and obsessive love. Although the characters have progressed beyond the socially contrived menstrual taboos that keep some men and women from sexual intimacy for a portion of every month, the author has, nonetheless, chosen to employ menstrual sex as a metaphor for the fatally wounded nature of the relationship. The scene in the hotel room functions like the scene in the tomb in *Romeo and Juliet*. Both couples end up bathed in blood. Shakespeare's marks the death of the lovers; Spencer's symbolically signals the emotional death that is pending.

There are many layers of meaning embedded in these menstrual transactions. In all four of the novels menstrual sex is associated with some sort of transgression. In Spencer's case, the young lovers have been forbidden to see each other; David is under a restraining order to stay away from Jade. In Malamud's case his protagonist tries *not* to transgress against the menstrual taboo and is subjected to a greater transgression—the political system's violation of basic human dignity. And Roth's characters, who gleefully see themselves as sexual outsiders, even sexual outlaws, engage in menstrual sex precisely *because* it is transgressive. Although for many people sex during menstruation merely requires some small effort in attending to its messiness, for these novelists it signals the messiness of human relations, the messiness of sexual desire, and, in Malamud's case, the messiness of ethnic identity and politics. Herein lies the irony in all three examples. Though each author seems to violate a taboo by even including menstrual references in his work, he nonetheless reinforces the taboo by associating menstruation with frightening or upsetting outcomes.

One additional novel deserves attention in this discussion, James Joyce's *Ulysses* (1914). Though Joyce does not include a specific menstrual sex encounter like those just mentioned, a brief moment in the midst of Molly Bloom's rambling 45 page soliloquy offers a woman's view (albeit written by a man) of how men rationalize having intercourse with a menstruating woman (the spelling and style are as they appear in the text and are intended to reflect the stream-of-conscious reflections of the character):

> ... I wish he had what I had then hed boo I bet the cat itself is better off than us have we too much blood up in us or what O patience above its pouring out of me like the sea anyhow he didn't make me pregnant as big as he is I don't want to ruin the clean sheets the clean linen I wore brought it on too damn it damn it and they always want to see a stain on the bed to know youre a virgin for them all that's troubling them

they're such fools too you could be a widow or divorced 40 times over a daub of red ink would do or blackberry juice no thats too purply O Jamesy let me up out of this pooh sweets of sin whoever suggested that business for women what between cloths and cooking and children… (p. 769)

Is imagining that the blood is from a ruptured hymen a way of denying contact with menses? Is the taboo so strong that men have to engage in a convoluted self-deception in order to satisfy their sexual desire? It's an intriguing question, one that is at the heart of many of the menstrual transactions throughout history.

References

Atwood, M. (1985). *The handmaid's tale*. New York, NY: Fawcett Press.

Burgess, A. (1962). *A clockwork orange*. London: William Heinemann.

Conrad, J. (1899). *Heart of darkness and the secret sharer*. New York, NY: Signet Classic.

Crane, S. (1990). *The red badge of courage*. New York, NY: Dover.

Curnut, K. (Ed.). (2018). American literature in transition, 1970-1980. Cambridge, UK: Cambridge UP.

Dollimore, J. (2001). *Sex, literature and censorship*. Cambridge, MA: Polity Press.

Fromm, E. (1941). *Escape from freedom*. New York, NY: Henry Holt.

Hawthorne, N. (1837). Dr. Heidegger's experiment. Retrieved on July 3, 2017 from http://www.hawthorneinsalem.org/mirror_eldritch/dhe.html

Hemingway, E. (1952). *The old man and the sea*. New York, NY: Charles Scribner's Sons.

Huxley, A. (1932). *Brave new world*. London: Chatto & Windus.

Joyce, J. (1914). *Ulysses*. New York, NY: Vintage Books.

King, S. (1974). *Carrie*. New York, NY: Doubleday.

Malamud, B. (1966). *The fixer*. New York, NY: Farrar Straus & Giroux.

Malamud, B. (1982). *The fixer*. New York: Washington Square Press.

Medoro, D. (2001). *The bleeding of America: Menstruation as symbolic economy in Pynchon, Faulkner, and Morrison*. New York, NY: Praeger.

Miller, W. (1997). *The anatomy of disgust*. Cambridge, MA: Harvard University Press.

Nussbaum, M. (2006). *Hiding from humanity: Disgust shame and the law*. Princeton, NJ: Princeton University Press.

Orwell, G. (1949). *1984*. New York: Harcourt Brace Jovanovich.

Patchett, A. (1992). *The patron saint of liars*. New York, NY: Harper Collins.

Patchett, A. (2011). *State of wonder*. New York, NY: Harper Collins.

Postman, N. (1985). *Amusing ourselves to death*. New York, NY: Viking Press.

Roth, P. (1995). *Sabbath's theater*. New York, NY: Simon & Schuster.

Roth, P. (2001). *The dying animal*. New York, NY: Simon & Schuster.

Skinner, B. F. (1948). *Walden II*. New York, NY: Hackett.

Spencer, S. (1979). *Endless love*. New York: HarperCollins.
Wells, H. G. (1895). *The time machine*. London: William Heinemann.

A Selective Catalog of Menstrual Transactions

The following list of nearly 40 titles is meant to give a glimpse of the range of authors who have made some use of menstrual references, either literally or in a symbolic sense, in their work. The list is far from comprehensive and readers are encouraged to add their own nominations to this menstrual canon.

Achebe, Chinua. (1959). *Things Fall Apart*. New York: Anchor Books.
Atwood, Margaret. (1985). *The Handmaid's Tale*. New York: Fawcett Crest.
Blume, Judy. (1970). *Are You There, God? It's Me, Margaret*. New York: Bantam Doubleday Dell.
Blume, Judy. (2015). *In the Unlikely Event*. New York: Vintage Books.
Coetzee, J. M. (1980). *Waiting for the Barbarians*. New York: Penguin.
Crane, Stephen. (1990). *The Red Badge of Courage*. New York: Dover.
Diamant, Anita. (1997). *The Red Tent*. New York: Picador.
Dumas fils, Alexandre. (1848). *Camille (The Lady of the Camillias)*. (Translated by Sir Edmond Grosse). New York: Signet Classics.
Dunant, Sara (1998). *Transgressions*. New York: Random House.
Eugenides, Jeffrey. (2002). *Middlesex*. New York: Farrar, Straus & Giroux.
Ferrante, Elena. (1999). *Troubling Love*. (Translated from the Italian by Ann Goldstein). New York: Europa Editions.
Heller, Joseph. (1966). *Something Happened*. New York: Simon & Schuster.
Hemingway, Ernest. (1952). *The Old Man and the Sea*. New York: Charles Scribner's Sons.
Hiaasen, Carl. (1991). *Native Tongue*. New York: Fawcett Crest.
Irving, John. (1985). *The Cider House Rules*. New York: Ballantine Books.
Jong, Erica. (1973). *Fear of Flying*. New York: New American Library.
Jong, Erica (1984). *Parachutes & Kisses*. New York: Penguin.
Joyce, James. (1922). *Ulysses*. London: Sylvia Beach.
Kaufman, Sue. (1967). *Diary of a Mad Housewife*. New York: Thunder Mouth Press.
Levi, Carlo. (1947). *Christ Stopped at Eboli*. (Translated from the Italian by Frances Frenaye). New York: Farrar, Straus & Giroux.
Levin, Ira. (1967). *Rosemary's Baby*. New York: Random House.
Lorde, Audre. (1997). *Zami: A New Spelling of My Name*. Freedom, CA: The Crossing Press.
Malamud, Bernard. (1966). *The Fixer*. New York: Simon & Schuster.
McCoy, Horace. (1935). *They Shoot Horses, Don't They?* New York: Avon Books.
Morrison, Toni. (1970). *The Bluest Eye*. New York: Holt, Rinehart and Winston.
Murakalmi, Haruki. (1987). *The Wind-Up Bird Chronicle*. New York: Vintage Books.
Oates, Joyce Carol. (2003). *The Tattooed Girl*. New York: Harper Collins.
Ondaatje, Michael. (1992). *The English Patient*. New York: Vintage Books.

Proulx, Annie. (1999). *"Pair a Spurs," Close Range*. London: Forth Estate. (originally published in the *New Yorker* magazine.)

Pynchon, Thomas. (2009). *Inherent Vice*. New York: Penguin.

Rabb, Margo. (2007). *Cures for Heartbreak*. New York: Delacorte Press.

Roche, Charlotte. (2008). *Wetlands*. New York: Grove Press.

Sedaris, David. (1997). *Naked*. New York: Little, Brown and Company.

Shaffer, Mary Ann, and Annie Barrows. (2009). *The Guernsey Literary and Potato Peel Pie Society*. New York: Dial Press.

Smith, Betty. (1943). *A Tree Grows in Brooklyn*. New York: Harper & Brothers.

Updike, John. (1984). *The Witches of Eastwick*. New York: Alfred A. Knopf.

Updike, John. (2009). *The Widows of Eastwick*. New York: Ballantine Books.

Welsh, Irvine. (1994). *The Acid House*. New York: W. W. Norton.

Yates, Richard. (1961). *Revolutionary Road*. New York: Vintage Books.

PART II

Mediating the Menstrual Landscape

This section consists of six chapters that explore the ways that menstrual transactions have appeared across a variety of mainstream media, beginning with a look at the appearance of menstrual elements in literary fiction with a close look at how several novelists have dealt with issues involving menstruation and sex, examinations of two menstrual dystopian novels as well as a glance at the appearance of menstruation in an early form of underground pornography. It then proceeds to the history of menstrual references in broadcast television. The chapters then move on to menstruation in feature films, including a snapshot catalog of over 100 films that employed menstrual elements in the stories. There follows a discussion of menstrual product advertising and how those practices have changed in response to changes in social circumstances, and then a discussion of how references to menstrual themes have appeared in the lyrics of popular songs. The chapters proceed with a look at what I refer to as "menstrual mischief," how the period has been politicized or employed to manipulate others or to reverse the negative attitudes that sometimes appear regarding menstruation. The discussion includes mention of four parodies of menstrual product ads that serve to challenge the assumptions customarily employed in those productions. The concluding chapter gathers together a random set of menstrual observations including a movie review, thoughts on women boxing and bleeding, patriotism and the period, and even a cameo appearance by Mel Gibson.

CHAPTER FIVE

Seeing Red on TV

Archie Bunker's Dilemma

In a 1972 episode of *All in the Family* Archie was faced with an unfamiliar experience, his wife's menopause. He is flummoxed and complains, "This change of life is a lousy thing, y' know. A man ain't got any say in it at all." At all other times—and on all other topics—Archie feels free to hold forth without restraint. But Archie is in this regard an "Everyman" whose understanding of the menstrual cycle and ability to talk about it are severely muted or strained.

Before Archie Bunker, as far as TV representations were concerned, there were no dads or husbands who had ever had a menstrual encounter. Neither Ralph Kramden of *The Honeymooners* nor *The Life of Riley*'s Riley nor *The Adventures of Ozzie and Harriet*'s Ozzie Nelson nor *Father Knows Best*'s Jim Anderson seemed to know a thing about the period. Perry Mason won court trials but never bought a box of tampons. Sgt. Joe Friday investigated missing persons and missing purses but never a missed period. For decades of television history the women on the air from Della Street and Margo Lane to Alice Kramden and Lucy Ricardo were period-free. That began to change once *All in the Family* arrived.

Aside from the occasional announcement of pregnancy, in effect an implied mention that a period has *not* appeared, the earliest fully developed menstrual reference on television occurred in the January 8, 1972 episode of *All in the Family* (Styler, Zacharias, & Rich, 1972) that dealt with the onset of Edith's menopause and its effect on her husband Archie. (Note: episode titles and air dates for cited programs are identified at end of chapter.) In the decades since, the period has made appearances in many guises serving a variety of functions including as plot devices or to reveal character traits or as a means of exploring social relations and underlying values. And, of course, menstrual jokes about PMS or male discomfort in dealing with the period have occasionally appeared. However, any attempt to create a comprehensive catalog of the appearance of any social phenomenon or behavior in television programs is bound to come up short. There are no reliable indexes of images, tropes or themes in programming so collecting specific examples is a random process of conversations and "findings" by colleagues, fellow researchers, social media mentions, and even casual acquaintances. Furthermore, no sooner has one discovered a new menstrual inclusion than the next season of programs offers up a fresh detail. To make the effort even more complicated, the proliferation of an ever-increasing number of cable and internet-based programming makes it impossible to keep track of any topic, let alone one as marginal as a fleeting menstrual transaction. And it is rare that menstrual elements are the central concern of an episode, though that does occur at times as, for example, in *South Park, The Cosby Show,* and *King of the Hill,* and the *All in the Family* episode already mentioned.

Due to these considerations, the following discussion will focus on several recurring themes that have appeared and that are sure to occur again. However, the discussion does not claim to be exhaustive or to include all pertinent examples.

The episode of *All in the Family* cited at the beginning of the chapter is a good representative of the important place that program holds as a pioneer in broadening the range of permissible topics included in prime-time TV programming. Menstruation, like another of the show's taboo topics, race relations, was considered inappropriate for situation comedy fare. And just as the daring moment when the guest star Sammy Davis, Jr., kissed Archie Bunker on the mouth became a milestone in the history of TV's treatment of race, the depiction of Edith's menopause titled "Edith's Problem" (Styler et al., 1972) put the period on the map as well. Though there was a lot of humor involved in the presentation, it was based on some fundamental psychological and social presumptions, including Edith's fear that no longer having a period meant that she was no longer a woman and that she would become less sexually attractive to her husband. It also appeared that entering this new phase made her more assertive as at one point she responds to Archie with one of his own signature phrases, telling him to "Stifle" himself when she doesn't like what he's saying.

It might be said that *All in the Family* brought menstruation out of the closet, but doing so with reference to menopause was a safe way go. Edith was a comic character whose dithering was a frequent subject of humor, and there was nothing "sexy" about her style. Audiences had a hard time imagining Archie and Edith having sex. A more daring episode of *All in the Family* occurred four years later on December 18, 1976 when another significant menstrual topic was introduced, the impact of a late—or missed—period on a couple's relationship. Gloria's fear of an unwanted pregnancy leads to a confrontation with Michael, her husband, who, being a good liberal concerned about over population, had considered getting a vasectomy but had put it off. Gloria's missed period makes them confront the issue and calls for him to live up to his politics (Doran, Arango, & Bogart, 1976).

The episode concludes with the missed period having been a false alarm but also with Mike going ahead with the vasectomy, thereby putting two taboo topics on the agenda while at the same time eluding the possibility of having to deal with the question of Gloria deciding to get an abortion, a topic that was a major social and political concern at the time as the Roe v. Wade Supreme Court decision that granted women the Constitutional right to choose how to manage their own pregnancies had been decided only a few years earlier on January 22, 1973.

Over time, these topics and others have become more common; however, the values associated with them are still rife with social stigma and stereotypes. While the effects on Edith of the hormonal changes of menopause were played for laughs, the matter received quite a different treatment in an episode of *Law and Order* in 2003. The title of the episode says it all: "Bitch" (Chernuchin, Weinman, & Makris, 2003). The plot centers on a murder committed by a high-ranking woman executive in a cosmetics company. Her lawyer creates a defense around the idea of "Menopause Rage." The woman had been experiencing severe symptoms that are fully spelled out in the courtroom scenes when testimony is taken. She had been experiencing hot flashes, night sweats, vaginal dryness and her business acumen was so badly affected that her company was facing financial ruin. She had been prescribed hormone replacement therapy but, as the expert witness testimony concluded, this led to "frontal lobe deficits" that resulted in a mental state that qualified her for use of the "temporary insanity" plea: not guilty on account of menstruation (Chernuchin, Weinman, & Makris, 2003).

Consider another case. On the surface one might think that Edith Bunker in 1972 and Samantha Jones, the sexually adventurous, forty-something year old woman in *Sex and the City* in 2000, have little in common, but when it came to their responses to the onset of menopause, they had strikingly similar reactions, and their responses were played out through encounters with men. Edith feared that Archie would no longer find her attractive; Samantha feared that she would be unable to attract the young, hot studs who commonly sought her out, that she was losing her sex appeal. As a result she is seen having sex with a man she is not really interested in and staring at the ceiling with a look of boredom as he thrusts into her. When he finishes, he looks down under the covers and exclaims, "Either you're a virgin or Aunt Flo just came to town," and goes on to fret about the stain on his expensive sheets. Samantha mutters an apology, smiles happily to herself and slips out of bed as the voice-over narration reports that there's still plenty of sex ahead for Samantha as her menopause has somehow been delayed. Though there was no mention of the man's awareness of menopause or the possibility that such a condition would make her less attractive, none-the-less, the script clearly suggests that a menopausal woman is likely to find herself with fewer desirable sex partners once menopause has kicked in (Bicks & Anders, 2000).

The same fear was on display in a 1986 episode of *Golden Girls* titled "End of the Curse" (Hughes, 1986) when Blanch, the most sexually active member of the Golden Girls group, missed her period. Her friends thought she was pregnant and engaged in spirited discussions of how to raise her baby, including what college the child should attend. But when Blanch announced, "I'm not pregnant. It's worse. It's much worse," they think she is dying and begin to commiserate. Instead, she says, "I'm not dying, Rose, I might as well be. It is menopause. I wish I could die because as far as I'm concerned this is the end of my life." Vividly, the emotional link between having a menstrual cycle and being sexually attractive to men is displayed. The internalized identity shaped by the experience of being told, "Now you are a woman" upon the appearance of the first period decades earlier has come full circle. If having a period means you have become a woman, then not having one must mean you no longer are. Notably, the relationships between these women's sense of self worth that is wrapped up in having a menstrual cycle is based on their feeling that self-worth centers on being attractive to men. Though it might seem as though having a period is "a woman's thing," for these sit-com characters (and perhaps for many women in their audience as well) it is their notions of male values that determine the existential meaning of their reproductive cycles.

A 1990 episode of *Roseanne* (McKeaney & Pasquin, 1989) also involved mistaking the onset of menopause for a possible pregnancy as Roseanne, who apparently has a good sense of when her period usually begins, realizes that she is nine days late and is seen using a pregnancy test kit. However, in her case, unlike the more common treatment, she is not panicked at the thought of menopause. Rather, consistent with her handling of other disturbances throughout the series, she takes the change in stride and goes on with her life.

One more menopause-based plot line comes to mind from the series *Orange Is the New Black*. Set in a women's prison, each episode consists of stories set within the walls of the prison interrupted by flash backs to scenes depicting the lives of the characters prior to their incarceration. In the 2014 season a character who had been a tough, crack cocaine dealer is now the head of one of the prison gangs. In a flashback she is seen at the age of 52 when she realizes she is entering menopause. She is hanging out with a group of young hustlers in her gang when she discovers that one of them, a young man she had taken from a foster home and helped raise, has been dealing on the side and cutting her out of his take. To demonstrate her power and sexual dominance she takes him to bed in an act that plays as incestuous exploitation then sends him out to buy her a treat where she has arranged to have him killed by a corrupt cop who is in her pay (Hess & Abraham, 2014). Here, once again, the supposed link between concern over sexual vitality and the onset of menopause is enacted. This character is portrayed as especially evil, as though she were a spider that consumes her mate after intercourse.

Once Norman Lear left ajar the menstrual closet door in that Queens, New York neighborhood of the Bunker family, the period's emergence has been gradual but steady. The most frequent appearance has been a relatively benign and safe context, the many family-based situation comedy series that air in the early prime time hours and whose plot lines commonly deal with parent-child, sibling or peer relationships. The casts are invariably made up of parents and several children spanning an age range and gender variety that allows for stories involving a wide range of issues. If a series lasts for a number of seasons, viewers experience the growth and development of the children in real time, and many shows include a young, pre-pubescent girl. So if the series has a long run (and the more successful ones could be on air for years), it is almost unavoidable that the writers decide to include story lines that address concerns such as the onset of menarche with its attendant physical changes, that the real-life young actresses are experiencing themselves.

For instance, Rudy, the youngest daughter in the Huxtable family on *The Cosby Show*, got her first period when Keshia Knight Pulliam, the actress cast as Rudy, was eleven years old, having been on the show since the age of five. Similarly, Darlene, Rosanne Conner's daughter (in *Rosanne*) began to menstruate in Season 2 when Sara Gilbert, the actress, was 14, having been on the show for a year by that time (Myer & Whitsell, 1990).

By far the most common menstrual transaction in family-based TV situation comedies involves the father of a young girl who is experiencing her first period. It is an ideal means of demonstrating several of the essential characteristics of men in the role of husband and father on such shows: that though they are often bumbling and clueless about dealing with their children, especially regarding anything sexual, none-the-less they are tender, caring and supportive of their daughters as they mature, well demonstrated by Dan Connor's "Good goin'!" to his daughter Darlene (Myer & Whitsell, 1990). Little more is said but the depth of the love and support are clearly noted.

A surprising exception to the pattern is the complete absence of Bill Cosby's Cliff Huxtable from the episode of *The Cosby Show* built around the youngest daughter's first period (Gartrelle, Kimbrough, & Bowab, 1996). Given that Huxtable is a gynecologist and is always positioned as the quintessential understanding father figure, it is puzzling why he is left out. All of Rudy's concerns are handled by her mother who also has a brief menstrual transaction with a young male friend of her son's. She deftly deflates a snarky remark she overhears him make about his girl friend's "time of the month" before going on to comfort her daughter.

Sometimes the fathers handle their daughters' menarche less gracefully. Though he is a doctor and is seen shopping for menstrual products with his daughter, the father in a 2005 episode of *Everwood* (Cooper & Paymer, 2005) makes the mistake of telling her soccer coach that she is menstruating and the coach in turn blurts out to the team, "She's got her period." The boys then mock her which results in her quitting the team, telling her father, "They made fun of me for being a girl." But the day is saved when she decides to move on to participate in gymnastics and her father recognizes his error (Cooper & Paymer, 2005).

The premier episode of the series *7th Heaven* in 1996, a program that remained on the air for 11 years, included a menarche scene as a means of establishing a number of relationship back stories, including the tender relationship that the minister father has with his daughter Lucy. When she gets her first period she shyly lets him know and he reaches out to shake her hand and says he will pay for dinner for her mother and sister to go out to celebrate. She smiles then runs back to get a hug and kiss him on the cheek (Hampton & Weisman, 1996).

Seven years later in the same series Ruthie, another daughter, experiences her first period but this time the drama focuses on the relationship with her mother. Unlike her older sister, Ruthie prefers to be left alone and even rejects her mother's attempts to comfort her and the offer to have a celebratory dinner. It seems that in the world of *7th Heaven* it takes a tender man to welcome a girl into adulthood (Hampton & Mordente, 2007).

Then there is a case where a father goes out of his way to ease his daughter's transition. In a 2007 episode of *Californication* the father takes his daughter shopping for her first menstrual product. In the store he finds that there is only one box of the pads, but it is suddenly taken by a woman who is shopping with her husband. He nearly gets into a fight with them trying to get the box in his determination to take care of his daughter who stands aside looking embarrassed (Kapinos & Winant, 2007).

Another example of how a menstrual transaction can be used to demonstrate a male character's chivalric support for a girl's "time of the month" is found in a 1994 episode of *Beverly Hills 90210* when the character Dylan has taken his young sister

Erica to a swimming pool. He waits for her outside the locker room and when she doesn't come out for a long while he goes in to find her crying in one of the stalls. She tells him she just got her first period and doesn't know what to do, so he calmly tells her everything will be OK and takes her to an understanding adult woman who gives her "the talk" and praises Dylan for his supportive behavior (Melman & Lange, 1994).

First period scenes that involve dramatic transactions between a young girl and a male character are not limited to father-daughter relationships. Even more problematic and fraught with tension are those where the male is a friend, a brother or even a stranger. Perhaps the funniest and riskiest depiction of a close encounter of the menstrual kind, one that most fully captures how deeply fraught with awkward meaning menstrual transactions are, occurred in an episode of *Curb Your Enthusiasm* (David, Berg, Mandel, Schaffer, & Steinberg, 2011). The set up involved a girl selling Girl Scout cookies getting her first period standing in the foyer of Larry David's home while writing up a cookie order. Rather than dashing off to find a woman to "take care" of the situation, as depicted, for example, in *King of the Hill* and *Beverly Hills 90210*, the protagonist rushes upstairs to get a box of tampons that belonged to his wife (who has left him), and stands outside a bathroom door shouting instructions to the bewildered girl inside. As he has never used a tampon either he unwraps one and tries to figure out its workings by sticking it under his arm as he works the tubular applicator.

Apparently she knows what menstruation is but has never been told how to use a tampon or other product. The episode is extraordinarily daring. Even the simple detail of having an older man hand a young girl he just met a tampon is startling, given the depth of social taboos requiring strict gender separation in matters menstrual. But to have him stand outside the bathroom door shouting instructions from the sheet packed in the box about placing the tampon in the vagina while the girl inside responds with confusion and frustration is risky indeed. But the most striking thing of all is that while both characters find the situation awkward, neither one is overly embarrassed, particularly the girl who calmly announces, "I think I just got my period for the first time" (David et al., 2011). Though she has apparently received little education about the technology, she is fully aware of what is happening in her body and accepts the fact that the adult she happens to be with when it happens is able to help her out. The fact that it's a male, and a quirky older one at that, seems not to matter at all.

At the opposite end of the spectrum from Larry David's blithe handling of the Girl Scout's needs is a 1999 episode of the animated series *King of the Hill* titled, "Aisle # 8-A." The plot line involves the King family—Hank, his wife Peggy, and their young son Bobby—agreeing to have their neighbor's daughter Connie stay with them while her parents are away at a conference. Hank, a shy and socially awkward man, is at home alone with Connie when she gets her first period and comes to him for help. Hank panics and calls his mother for advice but is unable to broach the topic. Instead, he rushes her to the emergency room of a hospital where a nurse tells him to just get her some menstrual pads and "Please, don't try band aids." He takes her to a supermarket and sends her into the "feminine hygiene" aisle where she is faced with the huge array of choices and is unable to decide what to buy. Finally, Hank joins her where they select a product and return home. When Hank's wife comes home and learns what has happened she is amazed: "You went down Aisle 8-A?!?! We've been married eight years and you've never gone down 8-A!" (Testa & Jacobsen, 1999).

The contrast between these two shows, though both are generously exaggerated for comic effect, strikingly captures the range of attitudes and responses men might have when faced with unanticipated and unwelcome menstrual encounters.

Less common than menstrual transactions between girls and adult men that are dramatized on situation comedies and family-friendly series are those involving girls and their male peers. A notable exception can be found in a 2001 episode of *Degrassi: The Next Generation* titled "Coming of Age" (Cameron & McDonald, 2001). This program, broadcast in the kid-friendly after school time slot, works hard at providing positive role models and healthy social behavior. In this case the plot focuses on a junior high school student, Emma, getting her first period at school, unprepared for its arrival. She stains her light-colored skirt and rushes to the girls' bathroom with her best friend. The girls are scheduled to give a book report together in the next class. Emma has nothing to change into, so her friend finds a pair of gym shorts that are far too big for her. When they go to class and stand in the front of the room she has to keep tugging at her shorts. Two boys in the front row tease her and one says, "What's the matter? Did Emma pee her pants?" She lifts her head and replies, "No, I just got my period—for the first time. Menstruation? You may have heard of it, happens to 50% of the population. Perfectly natural, nothing to be ashamed of, isn't that right Miss Kwan?" The teacher smiles and nods while the boys shrink down in their seats, but Sean, a more mature boy Emma has been attracted to sitting in the back of the room, perks up with interest in her confident frankness. Viewers had been prepared for Emma's assertiveness by an earlier scene in which Emma and her mother were seen walking through a shopping mall eating ice cream cones where a leering man says as they pass, "Hmmm, I'd like to lick that." Emma shrinks away but her mother turns and confronts the man saying, "Don't you ever talk to a woman that way!" The scene acts as a role modeling moment for Emma who replicates it in her response to the teasing boys (Cameron & McDonald, 2001).

When it comes to addressing the taboos surrounding menstruation, depictions of menarche are relatively safe spaces. Menarche is seen as a rite of passage and is often devoid of any reference to sexual activity, reproduction or the capacity to become pregnant. (The same approach is frequently employed in schools where girls are taught about ovulation, fertilization and using menstrual products but seldom about sperm and intercourse.) It is rare in TV programs to glimpse any menstrual blood stains or an actual product, though *Degrassi* is an exception in both of these areas.

Dealing with menstrual transactions between adult men and women entails a very different set of issues.

Surely the most emotionally and socially freighted menstrual transaction concerns sexual relations during the period. Given the layers of religious, psychological, cultural, and aesthetic impediments that have been erected against menstrual sex, it is a wonder that it ever happens at all. In fact, it is testimony to the power of the erotic impulse and the willingness to defy conventions that period sex does occur. And while it is the very existence of the body of taboos and imprecations against it that makes for dramatic tension, at the same time, the collection of social restrictions explains why period sex had to delay its appearance on television until the arrival of the more open climate of cable and Internet media.

A clever way of raising the subject is via a plot line that involves a couple who are about to, or are at least considering, sexual relations but are prevented from doing so by the reluctance of one or both of the parties to cope with the presence of menstrual blood. One program that portrayed such an encounter was an episode of the HBO series, *Entourage*, in 2004 (Ellin & Farina, 2005). The plot involved a young man who had been away from his girl friend for a number of weeks and was looking forward to renewing their sexual relationship. Upon his efforts to move the evening's encounter toward sex, she hesitated then told him that she did not want to proceed because of her period. When he suggested that they engage in some other means of satisfying his desire, she became annoyed and accused him of only caring about his own pleasure (Ellin & Farina, 2005).

The next day when he told his friends of his disappointing night, they chided him, suggesting that her rejection was not really about her period but that she was probably involved with another guy. They went on to express some bits of menstrual lore, including a few somewhat positive notions: "You don't have to wear a rain coat" and "They're hornier" (Ellin & Farina, 2005). In this way the program explored the personal dynamics of menstrual sex without actually having the characters do the deed. It thereby, in an indirect way, reinforced the taboo. And it went a step further later in the episode when Ari, the lead character's agent, expressed disgust at the thought of menstrual sex adding that "I won't even fuck my wife after she's played tennis" (Ellin & Farina, 2005). Ari represents a particular male sense of squeamishness about women's bodies and contamination.

In 1988 an entire episode of *Married... with Children* (Spring & Cohen, 1988) was devoted to menstrual transactions, including sexual behavior. The show involved both of the adult couples (Ted & Peg and Steve & Marcy) as well as the two adolescent Bundy children (Bud and Kelly). The original name for the episode was "A Period Piece," but it was changed to "The Camping Show" out of concern that women might be offended by an explicit period reference in the title. The plot centered on a camping trip the families were taking together that required them to inhabit a small cabin together. In an imaginative use of the belief that women living in close proximity can develop synchronous menstrual cycles, after only one night together the three women awaken to find that have all begun their periods at the same time. However, each exhibits a different "menstrual symptom" with Kelly experiencing severe cramps, March having severe mood swings, and Peg becoming horny and sexually aggressive. To add yet one more stereotype to the sketch, a bear senses the menstrual presence and is attracted to the cabin (Spring & Cohen, 1988).

Peg's increased libido, brought on by her hormonal changes, is treated in a bemused but not negative fashion. Her husband Ted, however, is turned off by her randyness as though menstrual contact is clearly to be avoided.

Another exploration of menstrual sex and the range of attitudes and behaviors surrounding it appeared in the 2017 series *The Deuce*, a gritty HBO program set in the drug and prostitution saturated world of New York City's 42nd Street in the early 1970s (Pelecanos, Lutz, & Hall, 2017). The significant scene takes place in a coffee shop hang-out where a group of five or six prostitutes and their pimp are gathered. Another prostitute comes in and hands money to the pimp who looks at the amount and tells her, "You're light." She explains that it's because she has her period which leads to an extended conversation about the necessity to "double up on the sucks" and various methods of coping with the period while still plying the trade. One of the woman tells about her use of the sponge and the problem of getting it out. The explicitness of the conversation goes too far for the pimp who leaves the table to commiserate with his fellow pimps at the bar. The scene concludes with one of them observing that "Women just be mysterious," and another claiming to be comfortable with menstrual sex, "I personally don't mind a little ketchup on my hot dog" (Pelecanos et al., 2017).

It is both amusing and enlightening to note the variety of viewpoints captured in the exchange. The women have a practical, professional perspective about how menstruation impacts their income and the ways they ply their trade, and they share trade secrets with each other. The pimp, though his livelihood is derived from their being able to manage their periods so as not to lessen his income, does not want to hear about how they do so. But when he joins other men at the bar it turns out that a variety of views are expressed, including one man who likens menstrual blood to ketchup and his penis to a hot dog.

Probably the most vivid depiction of a menstrual sex encounter in a video series occurred in the final episode of the first season of the 2017 Netflix series *I Love Dick* (Gubbins, Schreck, & Arnold, 2017). Through all seven previous episodes the sexual tension had been mounting as viewers were relentlessly teased by the question of whether Chris, the woman who has become so obsessed with the aloof title character, Dick, that she has written him thousands of pages of love letters, will ever manage to have sex with him. Finally, as they embrace passionately, the two physical manifestations of sexual arousal become plot points. The dialogue is explicit in identifying both. As they grind against each other, still fully clothed, Dick mutters, "I'm so hard right now. You feel how hard I am?" Chris responds, "You make me wet. It's all you." Dick takes his hand out of her pants and discovers that is it covered in blood. The passion comes to a quick halt.

Dick retreats to the bathroom, closes the door, and stands at the sink scrubbing his hands. Chris calls out to him repeatedly and, receiving no response, puts on her coat and stumbles out the door. She is last seen with blood running down her leg as she walks down the long road away from his ranch (Gubbins et al., 2017).

This scene captures vividly the power of the menstrual taboo. Once blood appears, no words are spoken—nor need they be—for the two characters, and the viewing audience as well, to understand the implications. The woman's menstrual wetness thoroughly deflated the man's hardness. It turns out that when it comes to vaginal secretions there's Good Wet and there's Bad Wet. The incompatibility between a hard penis and a menstrual vagina was made as clear as though the voice of God, as recorded in the book of Leviticus, had come booming into the room to rein in the lustful couple lest they violate the ancient pollution prohibition.

As previously mentioned, changes in the media landscape from cautious programming practices of network broadcasting that aimed for the widest audience acceptance possible to the arrival of cable systems with subscriber based channels that were exempt from FCC regulations and licensing and then to Internet based material that can be completely eccentric and random there has been a steadily growing permissiveness regarding every imaginable kind of content. Of course, that includes treatments of menstruation. There are sites devoted exclusively to menstrual fetishes and menstrual pornography. And within the genre known as Webcast series, the topic of menstrual sex gets its share of attention.

A good example of this development can be seen in an episode of the Webcast titled *Brunch on Sundays*. It violates just about every customary notion of what a TV series consists of, from its irregular length (each episode is anywhere from 3 and a half minutes to slightly more than 5 minutes long) to the language and conversational topics. It features three twenty-something year old women who get together for brunch every Sunday and discuss the preceding week's sexual encounters as well as such topics as the pros and cons of defecating with the bathroom door open.

As they narrate their stories, the scenes quickly cut back and forth between depictions of the events being described and the restaurant where they are dining. An episode aptly titled "Period Sex" (Weitz & Stubblebine, 2018) opens with two of the women celebrating the fact that they both are menstruating as they joke about bonding and belonging to "The Period Club, The Period Pod, the Period Pad!" Quickly the conversation turns to the question of whether one of them had sex with a new guy last night despite having her period. The scene cuts to the couple in the bathroom and the man's discomfort. The friend is outraged about male squeamishness, "So this guy wouldn't fuck you just because you were bleeding on your period... guys want to watch all these bloody movies but then don't want to fuck you just because they'll get a little blood on their dicks; that's fuckin' gross" (Weitz & Stubblebine, 2018).

The conversation continues to explore other aspects of how they deal with menstruation and sex including mention of a variety or reactions they have had from men they've had sex with. The gist of the exchange is that a man's attitude about menstrual sex is a measure of his sexual appeal: "Is he really an enthusiastic sex servant if he isn't enthusiastic about period sex?"

The menstrual arc from the coy to the crass is clear. From the goofy, flustered Edith Bunker and her befuddled husband Archie, to explicit menstrual boasting about technique and preferences, it would be quite an understatement to claim that, "times have changed." The changes reflect a combination of forces: feminism's impact on gender roles and expectations; increased frankness about bodily functions and sexual behavior; changes in the media environment that have lessened restrictions on the permissibility of previously forbidden topics; proliferation of media access points so that audiences have been fragmented into a myriad of sub groups. All of these forces contribute to shaping the menstrual ecology, and like any ecosystem, they overlap with one another in ways that are fluid and unpredictable. For a more detailed look at the process, consider the following case study of a program that has repeatedly included menstrual transactions in its plots and as a means of revealing character traits.

South Park—A Case Study

The Comedy Central series *South Park* that premiered in 1997 and shows no sign of running out of steam is known for including a variety of controversial topics. Quickly following its debut, *South Park* became one of the most successful cable programs of all times. It has frequently garnered higher viewership than any other basic cable program.

It is notorious for skewering every conceivable social value and convention with particular attention to "political correctness" as well as the Catholic church, feminism, race sensitivity, political office holders, and even Mickey Mouse and Jesus—to name just a few of its targets. Despite the take-no-prisoners approach, somehow its creators, Trey Parker and Matt Stone, have managed to escape significant backlash or calls to boycott their sponsors (a popular tool in media politics), perhaps because the victims of their satire span the political spectrum.

Along the way *South Park* has included in its story lines quite a number of menstrual references, and, since the major characters in the show are, with few exceptions, boys and men, the appearances constitute detailed examinations of menstrual transactions and male menstrual ignorance.

A common conceit of the program is that viewing life through the eyes of a group of fourth grade, pre-pubescent boys provides insights into the follies of adults: the boys' parents, teachers, and other authority figures. For instance, an episode titled "Are You There God? It's Me, Jesus" (Parker & Stough, 1999) satirized the path-breaking kid-lit novel by Judy Blume titled *Are You There God? It's Me, Margaret,* which became known for its frank and sympathetic chronicle of a group of young girls approaching puberty and the occurrence of a first period.

Readers familiar with the famous novel will recall that, among the many pubescent concerns they have, the girls are anxious to the point of competitiveness about getting their periods, the crucially important indication that they are becoming women. They gossip and even fib about who "got it" first, and important story elements concern their school viewing of a menstrual education film and shopping for menstrual products. With this in mind, the *South Park* episode offers what might be seen as a raunchy version of Gloria Steinem's essay, "If Men Could Menstruate." The menstrual story line kicks off with Cartman, the obnoxious, totally self-centered boy in the group, announcing to the other boys that he has just gotten his period and has become a man. His description is graphic, "You see, there comes a time in every child's life when they grow up and nature takes its course by having you bleed out your ass for a few days every month." At first the other boys doubt him but when they ask a passing women what it means to have a period it seems that the explanation confirm Cartman's claim, "It's when puberty hits and you bleed, you know, down there." Not wanting to be left behind, they go home to examine themselves to see if they are "bleeding out the ass" (Parker & Stough, 1999).

It turns out that the reason for Eric Cartman's condition is a stomach virus that causes rectal bleeding; however, all of the boys are so envious of Cartman's new status as a pubescent young man that the rest of the episode is spent charting their anxiety at not also having blood coming from the ass and trying to find out what a period is and how to deal with it. One of the boys, Kyle, even lies about bleeding so he can have the status that it bestows. And the "Margaret" of the show becomes Stan who goes about his days asking adults to explain to him what "getting your period" means, only to be met with confusing or evasive answers. The adult who is usually the most helpful in explaining the mysteries of adulthood to them, Chef, sings a song about the period but it is of no help in dealing with Stan's fear of being left behind his menstruating friends.

Again echoing a scene in *Are You There God?* the boys go shopping for menstrual products only to become even more confused when faced with the plethora of products that line the shelves of the store. Kenny, the boy who dies in every episode, tries to follow the directions for tampon use and inserts it in his anus, causing him to eventually explode as he fills up with feces.

Finally, Stan becomes so frustrated in trying to get an explanation of what the period is and why he has not yet gotten one himself that he prays to Jesus for an answer. But Jesus, being a man after all, is of no help either. Finally, God intervenes and answers Stan's questions as well as telling him that Cartman really has a virus and Kyle is faking. The program accomplishes several of its satiric intentions by creating a parody of Judy Blume's novel and at the same time laying out the various ways the menstrual cycle continues to be a taboo topic that children have a natural curiosity about but that adults turn into a dark mystery, particularly for boys. I wonder how the designers of health education curricula and lesson plans would feel about showing this piece in tandem with the usual corporate sponsored "Becoming A Woman" videos that are the major source of sex education in most schools.

Menstruation was put to use again in a *South Park* script titled "Bloody Mary" in 2005 (Parker, 2005, December) for the purpose of comically lambasting the Catholic Church, Alcoholics Anonymous, and adult gullibility in general. Here the plot brought together Stan's father, Randy Marsh, who has become an excessive drinker, and a statue of the Virgin Mary located outside of a local church. The stature has suddenly started to shoot blood out of its backside. The blood is believed to have miraculous healing qualities and the statue quickly becomes a holy shrine attracting hoards who line up for a chance to have contact with the blood and be healed of whatever affliction ails them. Stan's father, who is usually portrayed as a gullible believer in momentary fads and fashions, goes to the site, is squirted with blood, and believes he is immediately healed of his alcoholism. Eventually the Pope is brought to the scene to render judgment as to whether the event qualifies as a true miracle. He stands staring up at its rear. After a dramatic pause, the statue spews several streams of blood into his face and down his vestments. However, the Pope's pronouncement comes as a disappointment to everyone. He declares, "A chick bleeding out her vagina is no miracle. Chicks bleed out the vagina all the time" (Parker, 2005, December).

As a result, Randy concludes that he wasn't healed of his alcoholism and is helpless to resist the desire to get drunk.

Part of the joke is that it's a stature that is bleeding, a truly miraculous occurrence, but the question of the orifice from which the blood flows becomes the center of attention. At a far deeper level the story pokes at the deep-seated distinctions that Christianity makes between arterial and menstrual blood. The former, as a Communion ritual demonstrates, is seen as sanctified and a source of miracles; the latter, emanating from a woman's vagina, is a waste product of no consequence.

Apparently, this act of menstrual sacrilege crossed a line with the Catholic League, an organization with the self-appointed task of defending the civil rights of members of the Catholic Church. According to an article in ADWEEK (Nudd, 2005), the League rallied its followers to protest the episode which led to a decision by Comedy Central to cancel a scheduled rebroadcast of the episode, to remove it from the schedule, and to scrub screen shots of the offensive scene from their web site. The outcome is testimony to the power of the Catholic League in policing representations of icons of the faith and to the power of menstruation to disturb social protocols.

Another *South Park* exploration of menstrual matters was embedded in a story line that extended over several episodes titled "Mr. Garrison's Fancy New Vagina." (25) It involved the sex change operation that the boys' teacher, Mr. Garrison, underwent and became Mrs. Garrison. Once the surgery was completed, the teacher reveled in the new identity in a shallow, stereotypical fashion, flaunting a sense of what it means to be a woman. Eventually Mrs. Garrison becomes impatient that she has not yet had her first period, the real sign of having become fully a woman. But when time passes and no period has arrived, she concluded she must be pregnant and proudly rushes to her doctor for an abortion, another marker of one's full womanliness. Upon being told that she cannot have a period and cannot get pregnant and, therefore, cannot have an abortion, she becomes outraged and indignantly demands, "Yeah? Well what kind of woman can't have abortions and bleed out her snatch once a month?! You made me into a FREAK is what you did! And I want you to change me back!" (Parker, 2005, March). Ensuing episodes chronicle Garrison's quest to find the missing organ and regain his forsaken identity.

At first there seems to be little subtlety in the heavy-handed ways that *South Park* treats the targets of its satire, yet the underlying questions of how the meaning of gender is socially constructed then internalized by people is laid open by plot lines such as Mr./Mrs. Garrison's sex change. In this case the menstrual transaction occurs within a single character. Another episode titled "Towelie" (Parker, 2001) illustrated the role women play in enforcing the menstrual mysteries by "protecting" boys from the menstrual facts of life. The opening scene takes place at Stan's house where the boys are hanging out together. Cartman discovers a used tampon in the trash basket in the bathroom and they ask Sharon, Stan's mother what it is. When she stammers and says, "…that came from me; just put it away," Cartman thinks it is an aborted fetus. The boys press her for an explanation and she struggles to distract them by saying, "Boys, that's a… feminine thing. Alright, it's a personal, woman thing. I tell you what: If you just drop the whole thing right now, I'll buy you that new video game console you've been wanting" (Parker, 2001). Her gambit works. No more is said about the tampon and the episode proceeds as though the peculiar encounter had never happened.

In another episode titled "Cherokee Hair Tampons" (Parker, 2000), as the title suggests, tampons became one of the central elements in the show. The target of the satire, one that the script writers returned to frequently over the course of the show's history, is political correctness and the liberal community's penchant for new food fads and romantic notions of "living naturally." The plot is built around a "New Age" store in town run by a woman named "Miss Information" who offers an array of products for natural healing and living more in tune with the earth. At one point two men who the customers take to be "native American people" but are actually the comic characters created by Richard "Cheech" Marin and Tommy Chong—Cheech and Chong—enter the store with a box of trash that they pass off as sacred objects created by "our people," including a wire coat hanger that they claim is used in a special ritual. They also have bundles of hair wrapped with beads and string in tubular packets that they claim are Cherokee Hair Tampons. The gullible adults are so thrilled to have access to such authentic artifacts of tribal people who are "close to the earth" that they eagerly buy whatever the two hustlers can foist off on them (Parker, 2000).

The script takes a clever turn at the point where commercials are usually inserted into the show. As the program itself is animated, the appearance of actual actors on the screen triggers the assumption that a commercial break is in the offing. In this case, the small drama being enacted involved a mother and daughter sitting on a swing outside a pleasant suburban home having an intimate conversation. The girl asks, "Mom, did you ever have one of those heavy flow days?" Her mother tries to ease her concern but the first hint that this is not the usual discrete menstrual product ad comes when the girl says, "But remember the movie *The Shining* when the doors are opening up and…" The vivid image from that Kubrick movie of a flood of blood gushing from an elevator is an unexpected association. The dialog takes a further turn when the mother tells her daughter she just needs a better tampon and asks her, "What's the most absorbent thing in the world?" The answer is, "Well, Cherokee hair, I guess."

At this point the mother holds up a box of the product and the video images cut to a series of the usual sort of tampon absorbency demonstrations moving past several shots of tampons lying in glass bowls as blue liquid is poured over them. The camera pans to a shot of a young woman with long black hair wearing a dress that might be described as an Indian design lying on her back as a beaker of blue water is poured over her hair. The next shot is a close up of a woman's hand holding a long bundle of hair tied together with red cord and a small set of beads while the voice-over extols the virtues of the product.

The ad concludes with a scene of the girl bounding out of the house and running up to her mother who is clipping flowers in the front yard. She exclaims, "You were right, Mom! All natural Cherokee tampons really did the trick." Her mother smiles and says, "And when you're done using them, they make a great toy for Jesse," as she throws on of the hair bundles to their dog to play with. The mock ad concludes with an announcer's plug in the distinctive stoner voice of Cheech Marin: "Let the mysteries and the wonders of our people, like, change the way you think about tampons" (Parker, 2000).

The primary target of this episode of *South Park* is what the writers saw as the tendency of liberals to romanticize native peoples and to find fault with critiques of modern medicine in favor of so-called "natural" or "alternative" health practices. As the show was aired in 2000 it preceded the slightly later rise in alternative menstrual products such as cups, applicator-free tampons, and reusable menstrual clothes and underwear. In this regard it was ahead of its time. And as far as the gendered element in the story line, the two hippie stoners who are taken for authentic natives derive as much of their authority from their gender as from their putative ethnic origins. Both the women and the men who frequent Miss Information's store are accepting of the claims the men make about the hair tampons they have to offer.

It remains to be seen if the *South Park* creators will find even more ways of holding up to scorn the menstrual mysteries that are still in place. But perhaps the following example of another take on the topic derives in part from that influence.

Menstrual Defiance on *Broad City*

As a new generation of women performers, producers, writers and directors find opportunities to have their voices heard, menstrual elements have become more common, more nuanced, and much more explicit. Programs like *Broad City* demonstrate just how far menstrual acceptance has progressed since the days of *All in the Family*. Not only are the lead characters in the program involved in frequent casual sexual encounters (the word "promiscuous" is no longer in use having been replaced by the term "hook ups"), but their periods are on display as well. What is most striking about the menstrual references is that they seem so casual, so lacking in the previous time's tendency to lower one's voice, glance around before speaking, and select euphemisms to cover any discomfort that the topic might elicit. Yet, behind the seeming "matter-of-fact" nature of the references there lies an "in-your-face" intention to defy the conventions of menstrual decorum. Perhaps the best example of these changes occurred in an episode of *Broad City* titled "Jews on a Plane" (Jacobson, Glazer, & Aniello, 2016).

The set up finds Abbi and Ilana, the featured characters, joining a group of other young people on their way to Israel as part of a "Birthright" pilgrimage. Before boarding the plane with the other travelers, the two young women are seen preparing for the trip, which included Abbi wearing a light-colored pair of pants with a bright red stain on the rear. She ties a sweater around her waist and explains to Ilana that she is carrying a condom-wrapped stash of marijuana within her vagina but that the appearance of a menstrual stain will protect her from the drug-sniffing dogs at security. Sure enough, a guard's dog makes a move toward her crotch, but when the guard sees the red stain, he pulls the dog away.

Then, in the middle of the flight, Ilana gets her period but does not have any product with her, having been required to send her over-stuffed bag to the luggage hold. And we learn that on the first day of her period she has a particularly heavy flow. They both walk up and down the aisles of the plane asking various women if they have a tampon. When Abbi sees a man holding a piece of pita bread he is about to eat, she asks him if she could have it because it would be good to absorb her friend's menstrual blood. He looks at it for a moment then relinquishes it; the thought of eating something that would also be a good menstrual pad has taken away his appetite for pita—probably for a long while to come.

As the plot unfolds, they become increasingly anxious and repeatedly say things like, "She's going to explode. There's going to be blood everywhere. It's like a bomb." As this is happening on an El-Al flight, they are mistaken for terrorists, tackled by the flight attendants, and the episode ends with them being interrogated by tough Israeli security guards as they try to explain their behavior.

This single episode puts on display the kind of menstrual strategy woman have learned to employ by exploiting the avoidance behaviors that men have adopted toward menstrual presence as well as the bonding that women experience around their menstrual cycles. Abbi and Ilana join in a mutual quest to address her needs and even in the interrogation scenes the roles are played out. Ilana is confronted by a male officer who is uncomfortable dealing with the facts of the matter. Abbi is questioned by an equally tough woman security officer, but when Abbi tells her, "I thought this was about the stash I have up my pussy…" and describes in detail the variety of drugs she is carrying, the officer slowly smiles and says, "You wanna know what I got up my pussy?" (Jacobson et al., 2016).

Women Calling the Menstrual Shots

Episodes like this one whose entire plot line turns on a menstrual complication are uncommon. More often, there are simply lines of dialog that serve to reveal a nuance of a relationship, to display a character's personality or just to make a joke or wisecrack. Regardless of whether the menstrual transactions seen on television programs involve the onset of menstruation (menarche), the cessation of menstruation (perimenopause and menopause), the interruption of menstruation (pregnancy) or direct involvement with menstruation (menstrual sex or shopping for product), male presence in the matter is predictably dramatic and often a cause of tension. In other words, an excellent source of drama. Be it comedy, conflict, character revelation or simply a convenient plot device, menstrual transactions have steadily taken on a significant role in TV programming. And in doing so in ways that are sometimes subtle and sometimes "in your face" they have contributed to reshaping the core of beliefs and practices surrounding the most essential distinguishing gender marker that exists. It is not merely that the subject of menstruation is present in these programs. What's noteworthy is that in each one the emphasis is on male attitudes, behaviors and reactions.

Another way of looking at the reasons that depictions of menstrual relationships have changed over time is to note the identity of those who write, direct, and produce the programs. Unlike the earliest efforts to delve into menstrual relations that were largely products of male writers and producers (e.g. *South Park, Married with Children, All in The Family,* etc.), the five more recent programs with the most explicit and insightful perspectives have all been shaped or strongly influenced by women. Two are based on novels by women writers, *The Handmaid's Tale* by Margaret Atwood and *I Love Dick* by Chris Kraus, which also credits two women, Sarah Gubbins and Jill Soloway as creators of the series; two were created by women writers, *Broad City* by Ilana Glazer and Abbi Jocobson and *Brunch on Sundays* by Chris Pindalla, Shira Weitz and Haley Turner; and *The Duce* features and is co-produced by a woman, Maggie Gyllenhaal. Surely, the inclusion of women's insights into the topic has led to more nuanced outcomes. Coverage has widened to include topics such as the relation between menstruation and sexual practices, the logistics of "heavy flow" management, product availability, physical discomfort, and related subjects. It's hard to resist a pun by noting, now that women are involved, the catamenial is out of the bag.

Television Program References

Note: The following listing identifies the names of the programs, episodes and dates of broadcast of the shows discussed in this chapter. All of the programs were produced in the United States. While television programs that are aired on a weekly basis on traditional broadcast outlets have an initial date of screening, the fact that they are often rebroadcast and syndicated at later dates makes it difficult to identify when they actually enjoyed their largest audience or had their greatest impact. Furthermore, the fact that programs that appear on Web-based systems such as Netflix or Amazon are sometimes released all at once and accessed randomly by consumers further complicates the desire to specify viewing dates. These factors as well as the inconsistent way that production information is made available have resulted in some variations in citation content.

Bicks, J. (Writer), & Anders, A. (Director). (2000, July 30). The Big Time [Television series episode]. In S. J. Parker (Producer), *Sex and the City*. New York, NY: Darren Star Productions, HBO.

Cameron, T. (Writer), & McDonald, B. (Director). (2001, December 16). Coming of Age [Television series episode]. In L. Schuyler & S. Stohn (Producers), *Degrassi: The Next Generation*. USA: Epitome Pictures.

Chernuchin, M., & Weinman, R. (Writers), & Makris, C. (Director). (2003, February 26). Bitch [Television series episode]. In L. Carcaterra, M. Guggenheim, K. Johnston, & A. Zelman (Producers), *Law and Order*. New York, NY: Wolf Films.

Cooper, S. (Writer), & Paymer, D. (Director). (2005, January 24. Giving Up the Girl [Television series episode]. In T. Luse (Producer), *Everwood*. USA: Berlanti-Liddell Productions, Warner Bros. Television.

David, L., Berg, A., Mandel, D., & Schaffer, J. (Writers), & Steinberg, D. (Director). (2011, July 10). The Divorce [Television series episode]. In L. Streicher (Producer), *Curb Your Enthusiasm*. USA: Warner Bros, Domestic Television Distribution.

Doran, P., & Arango, P. (Writers), & Bogart, P. (Director). (1976, December 18). Gloria's False Alarm [Television series episode]. In M. Josefsberg (Producer), *All in the Family*. USA: Tandem Productions.

Ellin, D. (Writer), & Farino, J. (Director). (2005, June 5). The Boys Are Back in Town [Television series episode]. In M. J. Greenberg & J. Tashjian (Producers), *Entourage*. USA: Warner Bros, Domestic Television Distribution.

Gartrelle, G., Kimbrough, L., & Leahy, J. (Writers), & Bowab, J. (Director). (1990, November 8). The Infantry Has Landed (and They've Fallen Off the Roof) [Television series episode]. In T. Guarnieri (Producer) *The Cosby Show*. USA: Carsey-Werner Company.

Gubbins, S., & Schreck, H. (Writers), & Arnold, A. (Director). (2017, May 12). Cowboys and Nomads [Television series episode]. In J. Corey, C. Norris-Kahane, & J. Scheckel (Producers), *I Love Dick*. USA: Topple Productions.

Hampton, B. (Writer), & Weisman, S. (Director). (1996, August 26). Anything You Want [Television series episode]. In B. Hampton, A. Spelling, & E. D. Vincent (Producers), *7th Heaven*. USA: Spelling Television.

Hampton, B., Olsen, C., & Olsen, J. (Writers), & Mordente, T. (Director). (2003, May 19). Life and Death Part 2 [Television series episode]. In T. Mordente, C. Olsen, J. Olsen, & G. M. Patterson (Producers), *7th Heaven*. USA: Spelling Television.

Hess, S. (Writer), & Abraham, P. (Director). (2014, June 6). It Was the Change [Television series episode]. In T. Hermann (Producer), *Orange Is the New Black*. USA: Lionsgate Television.

Hughes, T. (Writer & Director). (1986, September 27). End of the Curse [Television series episode]. In T. Grossman & K. Speer (Producers), *Golden Girls*. USA: Touchstone Television.

Jacobson, A., & Glazer, I. (Writers), & Aniello, L. (Director). (2016, April 20). Jews on a Plane [Television series episode]. In R. Cunningham, K. Kiley, & R. McCormik, & J. Skidmore (Producers), *Broad City*. USA: 3 Arts Entertainment.

Kapinos, T. (Writer), & Winant, S. (Director). (2007, October 29). The Last Waltz [Television series episode]. In L. Fusaro (Producer), *Californication*. USA: Totally Commercial Films.

Melman, L. (Writer), & Lange, M. (Director). (1994, January 12). Thicker Than Water [Television series episode]. In P. Waigner (Producer), *Beverly Hills 90210*. USA: 90210 Productions.

McKeaney, G. (Writer), & Pasquin, J. (Director). (1989, February 14). Nightmare on Oak Street [Television series episode]. In L. Gelman, D. Jacobson, & G. S. Maffeo (Producers), *Roseanne*. USA: The Carsey-Werner.

Myer, B. (Writer), & Whitesell, J. (Director). (1990, September 18). The Test [Television series episode]. In J. Abugov, T. Arnold, R. Barr, & A. Lowenstein (Producers), *Roseanne*. USA: The Carsey-Werner.

Parker, T. (Writer), & Stough, E. (Director). (1999, December 29). Are You There God? It's Me, Jesus [Television series episode]. In A. Garefino, D. Liebling, T. Parker, & M. Stone (Producers), *South Park*. USA: Braniff.

Parker, T., & Stone, M. (Creators), & Parker, T. (Writer &Director). (2005, December 7). Blood Mary [Television series episode]. In F. C. Agnone II (Producer), *South Park*. USA: Braniff.

Parker, T. (Writer & Director). (2005, March 9). Mr. Garrison's Fancy New Vagina [Television series episode]. In F. C. Agnone II (Producer), *South Park*. USA: Braniff.

Parker, T., & Stone, M. (Creators), & Parker, T. (Writer & Director). (2001, August 8). Towelie [Television series episode]. In T. Parker & M. Stone (Producers), *South Park*. USA: Braniff.

Parker, T. (Writer & Director). (2000, June 28). Cherokee Hair Tampons [Television series episode]. In A. Garefino, D. Liebling, T. Parker, & M. Stone (Producers), *South Park*. USA: Braniff.

Pelecanos, G., & Lutz, L. (Writers), & Hall, A. (Director). (2017, October 1). I See Money [Television series episode]. In M. Gyllenhaal & M. H. Johnson (Producers), *The Deuce*. USA: HBO Enterprises.

Spring, S., & Vosburgh, M. (Writers), & Cohen, G. (Director). (1988, December 11). A Period Piece [Television series episode]. In S. Sprung & M. Vosburgh (Producers), *Married ... with Children*. USA: Columbia Pictures Television.

Styler, B., & Zacharias, S. (Writers), & Rich, J. (Director). (1972, January 8). Edith's Problem [Television series episode]. In N. Lear (Producer), *All in the Family*. USA: Tandem Productions.

Testa, G. (Writer), & Jacobsen, A. (Director). (1999, November 14). Aisle 8-A [Television series episode]. In J. A. Boucher & J. Dauterive (Producers), *King of the Hill*. USA: 3 Arts Entertainment.

Weitz, S. (Creator, Writer & Producer), & Stubblebine, V. (Director). (2018). Period Sex. In *Brunch on Sunday*. Retrieved on November 5, 2018 from https://www.youtube.com/watch?v=t56ljDaWjV8

Reference

Nudd, T. (2005, December 30). Catholics fight back against episode of "South Park." *ADWEEK*. Retrieved July 12, 2018, from https://www.adweek.com/creativity/catholics-fight-back-against-episode-south-park-19735/

CHAPTER SIX

Blood on the Screen

Menstrual Features

A credible argument can be made that many incidents of bleeding in film, literature, art and other modes of fictive or imagistic expression are actually symbolic references to menstruation, whether the creator or the audience is conscious of their presence or not. Several times in this book I have made that argument, for example concerning male novelists. Such occurrences have been called "vicarious menstruation" (Delaney, Lupton, & Toth, 1976) or even "menstrual envy" and I find such analyses frequently persuasive. However, in order to limit the scope of this chapter, which would become endless were it to attempt to cover all kinds of cinematic blood-letting, I have chosen to focus, for the most part, on those films with scenes that make specific menstrual references and that include male involvement in some sort of transaction concerning the presence of menstrual blood, paraphernalia or simply spoken references. Exceptions to this limitation occur when the symbolic implications are unavoidable. I have also limited the discussion to English language films and a very few others that have received wide distribution.

Only 30 films that include menstrual elements are discussed in any detail. That is a small, selective sample of those that exist. The intention is to create a framework for thinking about the complexity of the topic.

At the distance of more than 50 years after its release, it is hard to fully appreciate the impact and significance of *To Sir, with Love*—both book (Braithwait,

1959) and film (Clavell, 1967)—for its racial impact and to see how badly flawed both versions are. The main character has a strong strain of misogyny and a snotty air of class prejudice, though he also comes across as a race hero. The film follows the main plot of the novella, although it eliminates the inter-racial sexual and romantic relationship between the black teacher and a white, Jewish co-worker. Hollywood wasn't ready to take that risk yet. It even includes a key menstrual detail. However, while the novel spells it out explicitly, the movie ducks around the topic, leaving it up to the viewer's imagination to figure out what's going on.

Because the film industry has often relied upon novels as source material, menstrual details that first appeared in books were among the first to show up on screen. Adapting literary material makes it possible to include details that might otherwise be considered too delicate or offensive for the movie audience. Producers can simply respond to criticism by saying, "It's in the book! We're just respecting the author's work." A film is thus elevated in status to that of the higher-ranking book world and the audience is able to say, "No, but I saw the movie." Within a few years of *To Sir* three more films with menstrual details that were based on successful novels were released. Two of them, *The Fixer* and *They Shot Horses, Don't They?*, were adaptations of "serious" novels with literary aspirations and the other, *Rosemary's Baby*, was Roman Polanski's adaptation of Ira Levin's gothic novel of the preceding year.

In 1967 *To Sir, with Love* followed nearly in lock-step right down to much of the dialogue, the autobiographical novella. However, the menstrual detail is so obscured that audience members unfamiliar with the book were hard pressed to notice the significance of the veiled mention of a bloody sanitary napkin and its crucial role in revealing the protagonist's character and in shaping the plot. Even writers interested in the cultural history of menstruation have not noted its presence. The scene involved the fledgling teacher discovering a used menstrual pad smoldering in the heater in his classroom and causing a stench. He becomes so outraged, and assuming that the prank was done by a girl, he berates the girls and decides that hence forth the boys are to be called by their last names, the girls with the title "Miss," and that he is to be referred to as "Sir," hence the title of the story. His unwelcome encounter with the menstrual product requires him to assert his masculinity and insist on rigid adherence to gender labeling and behavior. There ensues a series of challenges, several involving the shedding of male blood—one in a boxing exercise and another with an accidental pin prick—that led to his fully realized manhood by the end of the narrative.

Immediately following *To Sir, with Love* there were several more menstrual film references, and they too were based on adaptations from successful novels. Both *The Fixer* and *Rosemary's Baby* used menstrual details as plot devices. In

The Fixer the protagonist's decision to decline a sexual invitation because the woman is menstruating has dire consequences, and the suspense in *Rosemary's Baby* is heightened by waiting for her *not* to have a period so the pregnancy story can unfold. *They Shoot Horses, Don't They?*, also following a detail from the 1935 novella it is based on, depicts a woman who must quit the dance marathon in the early stages due to painful menstrual cramps. During one of the brief rest periods she complains, "I got the curse comin' on" (Chartoff & Pollack, 1969). The line is rich in irony as it turns out that all of the marathon participants do indeed have a curse comin' on. The event sinks into a dance circle of hell, and they are subjected to greater and greater degradation and misery as they are beset with the existential curse of being alive in the darkest days of the depression. Though the marathon continues for more than a month past this scene, none of the other women appears to have the same problem. The symbolic value of the menstrual curse had been used up.

In the next two years, both *Diary of a Mad Housewife* (Gilbert & Perry, 1970) and *McCabe and Mrs. Miller* (Brower & Altman, 1971) alluded to the taboo against sexual relations during menstruation. The McCabe scene is noteworthy for the power that accrues to the brothel madam (Julie Christie) because she knows how women employ menstrual politics. She convinces the competing brothel operator (Warren Beatty) that he should become her partner by explaining that menstrual knowledge is a necessary management skill: "How do you know when a girl really has her monthly or she's just taking a few days off? How about when they don't get their monthly… What do you do then?" Proof of Mrs. Miller's concern is provided later in the film when we see an eager young customer ask, "Who wants to be next?" and one of the prostitutes replies, "Don't look at me. I got the curse" (Brower & Altman, 1971). The scene confirms the "no menstrual sex" taboo and validates Mrs. Miller's authority over McCabe.

The issue of menstrual sex was also used effectively in *Diary of a Mad House-wife* in a key transaction between Teena (Carrie Snodgrass) and her lover, George (Frank Langella). George claims to be a free spirited, anything-goes, kind of guy while Teena is an overly regimented, constricted woman who is struggling to shake free from a husband who treats her like a servant. Given her busy social and domestic responsibilities, arranging trysts with her lover is difficult. On one occasion the following exchange takes place. The lines are taken directly from the novel:

Teena:	"Next week, I could see you early in the week because I'm due to get the curse around the middle of the week."
George:	"I don't mind that."
Teena:	"I do."
George:	"You would." (Gilbert & Perry, 1970)

His willingness to risk emotional involvement with Teena and his lustiness are expressed in his indifference to the messiness of menses. She, on the other hand, is tidy, well ordered and organized. Her refraining from sex during her period is a sign of her fastidiousness and lingering reticence.

But the sarcastic crack George makes about Teena's rejection of menstrual sex ("You would.") reveals that his seeming openness is also a posture he strikes to demonstrate his superior sexual liberation. His remark implies, "I'm more comfortable with your sexuality, your womanness, than you are because I accept your bleeding and you don't." However, the scene takes on new meaning later on when George and Teena break up and Teena "accuses" him of being gay, suggesting that his womanizing is actually a means of denying his homosexuality. Seen from the perspective of 1970, a time when homosexuality was still viewed by the psychoanalytic community as a pathology in need of treatment and a condition characterized by strong desire on the part of men to become or act like women, George's willingness to have menstrual sex is a way of suggesting his desire to be feminized by contact with menstrual blood. His insult masks his disappointment that she will not give him access to that part of her sexuality, and he pouts childishly at her withholding it from him, in spite of the fact that he has previously praised her for her sexual prowess.

It was not until the release of *Smile* (Dougherty & Ritchie, 1975) that a Hollywood script used specific menstrual terms ("sanitary napkin") and a brand name ("Kotex," which at that time was, for many people, virtually a generic term). The reference occurs in a gag that involves the head custodian at a high school that is hosting a teen beauty pageant. The janitor, a vodka swilling Eastern European, is perpetually worried about the smooth workings of the school's plumbing because he fears that the girls will flush their pads down the toilet. His every appearance shows him listening for clogged plumbing, and he has insisted that the pageant's male host read an explicit statement from the "Maintenance Director:"

"It is requested that the girls not dispose of their sanitary napkins in the commodes. Since there are so many girls in the hall and since a sanitary napkin is thick and difficult (embarrassed pause), well, just don't do it." In a later scene we see the janitor feeling the wall like a palpating physician as he mutters, "It's starting. The pipes are backed up. I can hear them moaning and grumbling. They are. There they go. They're fed up with swallowing Kotex" (Dougherty & Ritchie, 1975).

Though today the film comes across as a trivial and, at times, distasteful piece of work that warrants little attention, at the time of its 1975 release it strove to be seen as a clever satire of the beauty pageants and crass commercialism that the "counter-culture" atmosphere of the anti-war and women's liberation movements sought to attack. The blue collar, ethnically coded janitor, with his Eastern European accent, is meant to be seen as a down-to-earth, working class Everymen who, unlike the fumbling, clean-cut men in suits who think they run things, can talk about embarrassing topics while others blush and stammer. However, while the film grants condescending respect to this colorful codger, it uses his obsession with the building's invisible plumbing to point out the lack of concern among the girls for proper management of their own inner plumbing. The grumbling pipes symbolize the girls' general emotional instability, their tendency to get clogged up and erupt. And though no individual woman or girl in the film is identified as having her period, the lack of effective management of the emotional lives of the featured women characters leads to interpersonal malfunctions.

Smile thereby became the first in what has evolved into a long line of films that employ menstruation as a metaphor for a notion of women's unsettled and unsettling emotional state. It functions within the context of larger motifs in the film concerning women whose sexual desires and expression are apt to create problems for men. Obviously, the idea that menstruation is both personally and socially destabilizing, an unpredictable and powerful force that is a continual source of dismay to men, long pre-dates this film or the very existence of the medium, so it is not surprising to see its perpetuation once the social climate reached a point where menstrual references could appear in mainstream films. So it is ironic that while the film breaks down one barrier, the taboo against references to menstruation in feature film, it perpetuates a set of conservative values regarding how women should manage their periods: they must keep them private so that men are not made aware of or inconvenienced by their presence. If only women would dispose of the evidence of their blood flow in such a way as to maintain male innocence, life's flow would be smooth. The plumbing metaphor aptly embodies a full range of meanings—health, order, cleanliness, social well-being.

Without doubt, the best-known and most vivid film treatments of menstruation are found in the adaptations of Stephen King's 1974 novel, Carrie. There have been multiple Carrie adaptations including Brian DiPalma's original in 1976, a made-for-TV version for NBC in 2002, a 1999 sequel titled The Rage: Carrie 2, a Broadway musical adaptation in 1988 and an off-Broadway production in 2012. There are likely to be more.

De Palma's film broke new ground, just as King's novel did, for its explicit depiction of Carrie's first period in a high school locker room shower, blood running through her fingers, down her legs and swirling toward the drain in images that pay homage to those in the famous murder scene in Psycho.

As far as I have been able to tell, this was only the third feature film to include specific reference to menstruation after *To Sir, with Love* and *Smile*. And it was the first to actually depict menstrual blood on screen. As such, it represents a cinematic menarche, Hollywood's menstrual coming of age. However, the number of actual menstrual blood depictions remains small. There are similarly few images of menstrual pads or tampons and all are of unused items or just the packaging.

Carrie could readily be charged with misogynistic intent both for its voyeuristic treatment of the girls in the locker room and its suggestion that menstruation unleashes in women dangerously destructive rage, the ultimate expression of male menstrual anxiety. The locker room scene is the realization of a boy's fantasy. The camera slips around the banks of lockers catching girls changing clothes, toweling off from the shower and showing brief glimpses of breast and ass. It resembles the Internet spy cam soft porn sites that claim to show candid pictures of similar locales.

The scene with Carrie, the outcast, showering alone after the other girls have finished, is voluptuous. She passes the soap over her body, legs and breasts taking innocent pleasure from the warm spray and sensuous stroking of her own hands. Then, as she rubs the soap between her legs, her hand comes away streaked with blood and she shrieks in terror as she (and we) see blood running down her legs and puddling with the water on the floor. In panic, Carrie runs from the shower screaming for help towards the other partially dressed girls, obviously believing that is mortally wounded. Her bloody hands smear other girls and they push her back into the shower, pelting her with pads and tampons from the dispensers on the walls, all the while chanting, "Plug it up! Plug it up!" A young teacher arrives in a white gym outfit and Carrie clutches at her, leaving large blood prints on her short tennis skirt. In her fear and fury, Carrie, unaware of her telekinetic power, causes the light bulb in the shower to explode, a harbinger of her future ability to control both electrical current and physical objects.

The following scene finds Carrie waiting in misery outside the office of Mr. Morton, the Assistant Principal, while Miss Desjardin, the teacher, strides back and forth explaining what has happened. Miss Desjardin is oblivious or indifferent to the fact that there is a large bloodstain on her pristine skirt, but every time she passes Mr. Morton's desk he involuntarily glances at it, wincing in mounting discomfort. His unease is intensified by the teacher's description of the fracas in the locker room, her ruminations about how unprepared Carrie was, and her reminiscences about her own menarche. Her self-disclosures are nearly unbearable for him as he fidgets and fuses, trying to slip around the subject and becoming so flustered that despite repeated attempts he cannot get Carrie's name right.

At first glance his muddled manner seems like a general character trait, an example of the too easy cheap shot at high school administrators so often portrayed as bumbling and clueless functionaries. But we cannot know for sure if this man is generally this inept as we have not previously encountered him.

Rather, his unhinged condition appears to be a result of his encounter with the forbidden, mysterious menstrual blood. This is a case of TMI—"Too Much Information!" Consider the conditions of menstrual relations in 1974 or 1976 the respective dates of the novel's publication and the film's release. Imagine the discomfort level of a middle-aged high school principal having to sit at his desk while a menstrual stained young woman in a short white skirt parades back and forth describing her own first period and then having to deal with a frail and frightened girl whose menstrual circumstances he has just learned the intimate details of. Under the circumstances, his shaky poise is admirable.

Carrie was released only one year after the forgettable *Smile* and it is a striking contrast with it. It expressed the most terrifying of male menstrual anxiety and it was remains the most memorable and influential exploration of the topic.

Soon after *Carrie* Woody Allen released what some consider his best film, *Annie Hall*. The movie established a number of signature elements of Woody Allen movies including the neurotic personality of the recurring Alvy Singer character, and Allen's distinctive directorial style. The film was unique in many ways, including its casual inclusion of two menstrual references.

The first takes place outside a movie theater, an appropriate setting given Allen's interest in the relationship between life and movie fiction. Annie is a few minutes late for a date with Alvy, and when she arrives they start to squabble. He says, "Hey, you are in a bad mood. You must be getting your period," to which she replies, "I'm not getting my period. Jesus, every time something out of the ordinary happens, you think I'm getting my period" (Joffe & Allen, 1977). Alvy becomes embarrassed that she has mentioned her period loudly enough for others to hear and changes the subject. However, they are two minutes late for the start of the film and he refuses to attend. Just as "being late" is code for not having gotten one's period and, therefore, the fear of being pregnant, lateness for Alvy is a sign of his own insecurities, especially his problems with romantic relationships. (He makes the link later in the film in a sly though explicit reference to oral sex, one of the earliest in feature film, when Pam—the flaky *Rolling Stone* reporter played by Shelly Duval—apologizes for having taken so long to have her orgasm and Alvy rubs his chin and complains, "Yeah, I thought I was gonna throw my jaw out of joint." (Joffe & Allen, 1977)).

Twenty scenes after the first menstrual reference (about 40 minutes of film time), following another fight with Annie, Alvy steps partially out of character and strides down the street asking passing strangers how they manage their sex lives and relationships. Eventually, he ends up talking to a horse, telling it "When my mother took me to see *Snow White*, while the other kids were falling in love with Snow White, I was falling in love with the Wicked Witch." This leads to a jump to a surprising cartoon animation in the style of Disney's *Snow White* with Annie as the Wicked Queen preening in front of a mirror. They have the following exchange:

Annie:	We never have any fun any more.
Alvy:	How can you say that?
Annie:	Why not? You're always leaning on me to improve myself.
Alvy:	You're just upset. You must be getting your period.
Annie:	I don't get a period. I'm a cartoon character. Can't I be upset once in a while? (Joffe & Allen, 1977)

The scene is an example of Allen's fondness for violating cinematic conventions. In this case, suddenly finding themselves watching a cartoon, and a Disney-like one at that, the audience is given a break from the story line and invited to ask, What's the difference between a cartoon and a "live action" movie? Is there a difference? However, since the dialogue is nearly identical to the earlier scene, it forces the audience to review the content as well: how men and women relate to one another around the subject of menstruation. Are men somehow like simple, two-dimensional cartoon characters who insist on attributing to women biological reasons for their emotions, reasons that allow men to avoid emotional engagement themselves? And why *don't* women in films get periods, whether they are cartoon characters or "real?" The point of the cartoon inclusion is to suggest that perhaps there is not such a clear difference between cartoon characters and "real" ones, or even between film characters and actual people.

Allen has employed menstruation to point out how strenuously men work at enforcing the notion of difference. Given that *Annie Hall* is a heterosexual romance bent on exploring the nature of romantic relationships, menstruation emerges as one means of demonstrating how important the reinforcement of sexual identity can be.

The year following *Annie Hall* another film with aspirations to counter-culture status appeared, the musical *Grease*, starring John Travolta, fresh from his success the year before in *Saturday Night Fever*, and Olivia Newton John, at that time a rising pop music star. Like *Annie Hall*, *Grease* includes two menstrual references that are used to reveal character and theme. The first shows a boy secretly placing a menstrual pad in a girl's bag so that when she accidentally pulls it out, she shrieks, throws it in the air and runs from the classroom in shame. The second occurs when the "bad girl," Betty Rizzo (Stockard Channing), suspects she is pregnant and quips to a friend, "I feel like a defective typewriter... I skipped a period" (Carr & Kleiser, 1978).

The first detail, which happens early in the film, is intended to capture the ambience of teen culture during the film's mid-1950's setting, a time when any public acknowledgment that a girl might actually need a menstrual product would be cause for acute embarrassment. At the same time, inclusion of the boy's prank in the movie, though the pad is seen only fleetingly, is a way of saying to the late 1970s audience, "Look how cool and liberated we are; we can include taboo stuff in our film that no one in the 50's would have dared to do."

The "typewriter" joke with its actual use of the word "period," even as a pun, takes the ploy one step further. In all likelihood the audience (or a good part of it) likes and identifies with Rizzo more strongly than with Sandy, the Olivia Newton-John character, and appreciates her bold frankness. In her liberated, openly expressed sexuality she is the tough, assertive woman that members of the audience might aspire to become.

Though no men are involved in the scene when Rizzo makes her period joke, men in the audience might well hope that the women in their own lives would manage the fact of a missed period as Rizzo has—by keeping it to herself and not expecting the guy who "got her pregnant" to have any responsibility for the outcome. Thus, the film employs menstruation as a trope for demonstrating how times have changed over the two decades between the film's setting and its production, but also how much they haven't. For all its surface progressiveness, *Grease* is yet a cautious film. It might be silly and out-dated to shriek in shame just because people know you have a pad in your purse, but it's still a potential tragedy if you "fool around" and miss your period. Fortunately for Rizzo, and for the audience's presumed preference for a happy ending, she gets her period before the movie ends and everyone is saved from having to deal with the social consequences of an unwanted pregnancy.

At decade's end two more films that touched upon menstruation were released, both in the same year with strikingly similar titles: *An Unmarried Woman*, directed by Paul Mazursky (1978), and Wendy Wasserstein's *Uncommon Women... and Others* (1978), a made-for-TV adaptation of the Broadway play. Neither one included men in the menstrual material. In the former the lead character confides to her woman psychotherapist the details of her embarrassment at the time of her menarche, and in the latter the scene involves the moment when Rita (Swoozie Kurtz) boasts of having tasted her menstrual blood and goes on to tell her college dorm mates that "all men should be forced to menstruate" (Mazursky, 1978). The intimacy of these scenes is similar to the one in the somewhat later *Agnes of God*

(Jewison, 1985) in which the Mother Superior (Ann Bancroft) and psychotherapist (Jane Fonda) mistakenly conclude that the blood-stained sheets that Agnes is
ashamed of were from her period rather than the rape that took her virginity and
left her pregnant. Instances such as these gradually helped make it more acceptable to mention menses, especially in conversations between women in movies
aspiring to be seen as serious artistic expressions, but they mostly kept men out of
the picture.

In the early 1980's men began to have a higher level of visibility in the
menstrual lives of women in film. Two teen romance films, *Blue Lagoon* (Kleiser,
1980) and *Endless Love* (Lovell & Zeffirelli, 1981), illustrate the challenges that
were involved. Both were adapted from novels and starred Brooke Shields, and
both are significant as they represent contrasting views of the appropriate place
of menstruation in film. The film version of *Endless Love* is noteworthy for its
excision of one of the most vivid menstrual sex scenes in popular fiction just as
Blue Lagoon is significant for the addition of menstrual details that were not in
the original novel.

The novel *Blue Lagoon* is a simple tale of natural innocence originally published in 1907 by H. DeVere Stacpoole, a British naturalist who wrote about the
exotic environment of the South Pacific as well as fiction in the "noble savage"
tradition. He might be thought of as a romantic version of Joseph Conrad. The
book tells a story of two small children, a boy and a girl, who, along with an
old sailor, are ship wrecked on a beautiful desert island. The sailor dies before
the children reach puberty but not before he has taught them the necessary
survival skills to live comfortably in their Edenic setting. As might be expected,
on their own they discover sex and successfully produce a baby, though they
remain innocent of the links between their sexual pleasures and the outcome. All
of this is described with Victorian discretion and ends happily when they and
their baby are rescued after having been lost for more than a decade. Cinematic
tastes in 1980 required that the film adaptation include stars (Brooke Shields
and Christopher Atkins are flawlessly beautiful and always well dressed in dainty
loin clothes; Brook's flowing hair is just long enough to cover her breasts.). Less
subtle details of their sexual awakening are also called for. Therefore, we see
references, though not too explicit, to the boy's masturbation, to their pubescent
desire, and to their lovemaking.

The means of expressing the children's sexual maturity is to add to the story
a menarche scene for the girl and a symbolic menses for the boy. The girl's first
period occurs while she is bathing in the lagoon and discovers blood on her fingers
while she is touching herself. The scene is reminiscent of the *Carrie* scene in the
shower and the girl reacts similarly by screaming in panic. However, when the boy

arrives, she suddenly becomes shy and makes him go away. Later that night as they sit around their campfire, she refuses to answer his questions about what is wrong with her or to let him examine the "wound" from which she is bleeding. It seems that even in a setting free from society's taboos and conditioning, women still feel shame about their periods and instinctively shut men away from physical closeness or even knowledge of the menstrual mystery.

The next day while the boy is out on his skiff fishing with a string hand line, a shark latches on to his bait and, before he can control the line, pulls it through his hands causing deep cuts across his palms. He grimaces in pain and stares at his bloody hands the same way that the girl did in the lagoon. These two moments mark their transition into puberty and lead shortly to their sexual coupling. The most interesting aspect of the treatment is that the film seems to espouse the notion that for men and women alike, bleeding is part of becoming an adult. Though the boy's menarche is symbolic, it suggests the need for some kind of blood parity between the sexes before a stable adult community can be created, one that allows for shared sexual pleasure and its by-product, children. The fishing scene is strikingly (and suspiciously) similar to portions of Hemingway's *The Old Man and the Sea* in which Santiago undergoes an identical, though far more excruciating, ordeal during the prolonged male initiation rite he undergoes.

In the making of the film adaptation of Scott Spencer's 1979 novel, *Endless Love* a year after the release of *The Blue Lagoon*, Franco Zeffirelli was handed an opportunity to explore the place of menses in two characters' sexual encounters but apparently choose not to. It is not known if this was Zeffirelli's decision or that of others who shaped and financed the film, but the result was the elimination of a scene that is both startlingly explicit and symbolically central to the novel. It appears as though the director was trying to recreate in modern times and language his successful and beautiful version of *Romeo and Juliet* (Brabourne & Zeffireli, 1968) from a decade earlier. That film was highly influential, particularly for the casting of two young actors who were close in age to the characters they portrayed and for the sensuousness—even lustiness—of their adolescent desire. This was a far cry from the staid, ethereal love depicted by Norma Shearer and Lesley Howard thirty years earlier in the first sound film of *Romeo and Juliet* (Thalberg & Cukor, 1936). After Zeffirelli, an "older" actor could never again play a filmed version of any of Shakespeare's troubled youth, as ensuing productions of *Romeo and Juliet* and *Hamlet* have proven. The brief glimpses of Juliet's breasts and Romeo's ass were daring for the times and have continued to cause problems for teachers who use the film to introduce adolescents to Shakespeare.

The distance between Juliet Capulet and Jade Butterfield of *Endless Love* is not as great as it might first appear. Shakespeare lets us know that Juliet has begun to menstruate by the fact that her family has declared her ready to wed and by her mother's report that she herself had already been pregnant by the time she was her daughter's age. Scott Spencer's characters are as driven and compulsive as Shakespeare's, the difference being that the girl in the novel grows up and goes on to other relationships and an adult life while the boy stays perpetually at the stage of his adolescent obsession. In fact, he is so completely stuck that he enters a deranged state of arrested development, becomes a stalker and is committed to a mental institution.

As the 1980's progressed, two films captured the nature of the menstrual transaction and brought the topic into the open even further, much as Woody Allen did in *Annie Hall. Monty Python's The Meaning of Life* (Goldstone, Gilliam, & Jones, 1983) and *Sixteen Candles* (Green & Hughes, 1984), two ambitious social satires, employed broad humor to expose menstrual social conventions. The key scene in *The Meaning of Life* might well have been titled, "Penis, Puke, and Period." It sets out to poke fun at British propriety and the tendency to ignore even the most inappropriate behavior in the interest of social convention.

The setting is an elegant restaurant and we come in during the performance of a Noel Coward-styled lounge song about the penis. Due to the sophisticated style of delivery and the pleasant manner of the performer, the diners take no notice of its crudeness in spite of its graphic language. The second part of the scene features an immensely obese man who proceeds to devour everything on the menu and then vomit it over the table, waiters and adjacent diners. Throughout his disgusting sprays, the maitre 'd, played unflappably by John Cleese, continues to hover over him attending to his needs with British *sang froid*. As the vomiting proceeds, two couples at an adjacent table decide to leave. Though they are clearly driven out by the grossness of their fellow diner, propriety forbids that they say so, even when Cleese inquires as to why they are leaving. Rather than admit that anything is amiss, one of the women calmly explains that their departure is due to her period, an admission that Cleese takes in with the same equanimity as his handling of the puke fest:

Cleese:	Is there something wrong with the food?
Man:	No, the food was excellent.
Cleese:	Perhaps you're not happy with the service?
Man:	No, no, no complaint.
Woman:	It's just that we have to go. I'm having a rather heavy period.
Man:	ahem, … and we have a train to catch.
Woman:	Yes! Yes, of course, we have a train to catch and I don't want to start bleeding all over the seats. (Goldstone & Gilliam & Jones, 1983)

The juxtaposition of the three "unmentionables," penis, vomit and menstruation, creates a commentary on social conventions about permissible language and behavior, and the grouping of these particular three makes them comment on each other. The penis and period portions are about permissible language. The singer has not shown his penis and has sung about it in the most pleasant way imaginable. The woman has mentioned her period in a friendly, chatty manner as she would discuss the weather or her garden. However, the vomiting man has done something that is physically repulsive and sickening, yet no one makes the least distinction between words and deeds. Furthermore, the scene is artfully balanced with the penis song and menstrual mention framing the binge vomiting. Though I have not done comparable research on the frequency of penis references in film, it seems that both words are similarly uncommon so that the scene points out the universal squeamishness the public feels about mention of anything having to do with either sex's genitalia, even if expressed in the most benign or pleasant fashion.

The menstrual material in *Sixteen Candles* is much more fully developed than in any previous film. The film is modeled after 50's and 60's teen movies and TV family situation comedies like *Father Knows Best* and *My Little Margie*, and is set in an all white suburb with a traditional family of father, mother and three children. Paul Dooley plays the wise yet befuddled father, a stock character he has played in numerous other films. The main character is the middle child, Samantha, whose birthday falls on the day of her older sister's wedding and, as a result, is forgotten by everyone in the family. Within the first four minutes of the movie we learn that the oldest child is a young bride-to-be who has gotten her period on the day before her wedding. She has commandeered the bathroom, leaving her father in the hall with a mouthful of toothpaste, responding to his complaints saying, "I happen to be having a serious problem." Her eleven-year-old, wise-cracking brother says to his father, "Dad, she's getting her period. Should make for an interesting honeymoon, huh?" to which he responds, "Where do you learn this stuff?" He answers, "At school." Rather than being shocked at how explicit his son's sex education is, he sighs in relief and says, "Good. I'm getting my money's worth" (Green & Hughes, 1984).

This exchange encapsulates a significant change in film practice and suggests similarly significant changes in menstrual relations in general, including within family dynamics. It begins with the young woman's frank and matter-of-fact reference to her period. Though it is slightly euphemized ("I happen to be having a serious problem."), the boy gets the message right away and the father picks up the meaning once the son clues him in.

The movie continually shifts back and forth between homage to the 50s conventions and occasionally smug flaunting of its 80s coolness. We learn that not only is menstruation now in the curriculum, but that it has been released into the realm of casual banter. In an effort to relieve her cramps the bride takes too many valiums and is late for the wedding. Her mother explains, using a euphemism that was new to me, "We're sorry. Her monthly bill came early." The expression efficiently captures the mother's sentiment that there is a price to pay for being a woman. When they finally assemble in the anteroom of the church, the bride passes out near an open microphone so that the entire congregation hears the mother say, "Please be quiet! We don't want to announce to everyone that she's got her period." The topic gets one more laugh a few moments later when the groom jokes to the priest, "Guess those people who thought we had to get married are feeling pretty stupid right now." This is the only feature film I am aware of that uses menstruation as a running gag, although the TV show *South Park* has since done so repeatedly. By referring to the subject in four scenes and hinting that it will continue into the honeymoon afterwards, the film makers came up with a way of pointing out how much times have changed from those days of social amenorrhea when, for all we could tell, menstruation did not exist.

By the end of the 1980s menses had become an acceptable topic of at least glancing interest, especially if used for humor, plot advancement or as symbolic of some psychological or social condition. Then, in the mid-1990s, filmmakers began to explore the nature of the menstrual transaction with more depth and subtlety. Men, even boys, appeared to be more knowledgeable about menses and while some men were comfortable with the topic, others were even more overtly hostile in the ways they expressed their feelings and disgust.

The change showed up in five very dissimilar films released within a short time of each other: *Pulp Fiction* (Bender & Tarantino, 1994), *Tom & Viv* (Kass, Samuelson, Samuelson, & Gilbert, 1994), *Kids* (Vachon, Van Sant, Woods, & Clark, 1995), *Clueless* (Rudin & Heckerling, 1995), and *Your Friends and Neighbors* (Golin, Patric, & LaBute, 1998). Two of them deal with adolescents and three with adult men; the contrasts are striking.

Clueless offered a look at women's sexuality and menses that was different from previous Hollywood features. Cher, Dionne and the other girls in Beverly Hills are as open and comfortable as can be with their sexuality, including their periods, although the boys still have a long way to go. The film has two menstrual references that function much like those in *Grease* with echoes of *Annie Hall*. The first, early in the film, occurs during a spat between Dionne (Stacey Dash) and her boyfriend Murray (Donald Faison) when she accuses him of cheating on her. He counter-attacks by playing the menstrual card, "Why you gotta go there? Is it that time of the month again?" The other boys and girls gathered around gasp in recognition that the fight has just escalated. What makes the scene different from earlier movie transactions such as this is that the kids are indifferent to the public nature of the reference. Instead of being embarrassed at an allusion to her period, Dionne is offended that he would attempt to distract attention from his philandering by such a cheap attack. It is clear to everyone involved that he is in the wrong and that there is no merit in his desperate move. Menstrual instability has ceased to be a charge with any rhetorical power.

About an hour later in the film Cher too has a menstrual transaction when she successfully plays the menstrual card to her advantage. When she is scolded by her teacher, Mr. Hall (Wallace Shawn), for her tardiness, she explains:

Cher: I was surfing the crimson wave. I had to haul ass to the ladies.
Mr. Hall: I assume you're referring to women's troubles and so I'll let that one
            slide. (Rudin & Heckerling, 1995)

Cher tosses off her line about "the crimson wave" with insouciance in front of her entire class and no one takes the least notice. She knew she could play on Mr. Hall's gentlemanliness as well as the generational difference—he is at least 30 years her senior. Her manipulative use of a menstrual reference illustrates how easily she can manage men, especially older ones like Mr. Hall and her father, who are defenseless against the embarrassment they feel when confronted by a menstruating woman, or at least one who claims to be. Though Mr. Hall is not completely flustered and is capable of a mild rejoinder, his quaint language ("women's troubles") underlines the film's point about how young women and the times have evolved, including the menstrual ethos in which they live.

The kids in *Kids*, a film released the same year, are as savvy as those in *Clueless* but of a far nastier ilk. Unlike the sweet teens in the suburbs of Los Angeles who sometimes actually live up to the film's title, the boys who inhabit the streets of New York City are anything but "kids" in their quest for virgins to deflower and mischief to make. The menstrual detail occurs when two of the boys are rifling through the bedroom of one of their mothers looking for cash she has hidden away. The other boy comes across the woman's supply of tampons and unwraps one then takes it by the string and dips it into the glass of cranberry juice he is drinking. He holds it up and speaks to his friend:

"You ever take one of these things out with your teeth?"
"Steesh."
"Your girls don't bleed yet, that's why. My girl's got mad flavor." (He sucks on the tampon.) "Heavy flow." (Vachon et al., 1995)

He continues to dangle the tampon by the string and suck on it. The moment captures how jaded the boy is as well as how knowledgeable. He knows what the device is used for and is able to make a mocking joke about it. And the action, combined with the fact that his friend is stealing his own mother's money, expresses how far beyond the pale these adolescents are.

The three adult males in films of the same time frame exhibit different perspectives. Quentin Tarantino's *Pulp Fiction* included a line that economically captured a male perspective on menses and the fact that men had not overcome their disgust with it. Due to the accidental shooting of an innocent boy in the back seat of their car, Vincent and Jules (John Travolta and Samuel L. Jackson) are spattered with blood and must clean up both the car and themselves as well as disposing of the body. One of the differences in personal habits between Vincent and Jules is that Vincent is careless and sloppy about the small details of daily life (a trait that eventually costs him his life) while Jules is neat and fastidious. At one point Jules enters a bathroom after Vincent has used it and finds the place a bloody mess, including the towel. When he criticizes Vincent for his slovenliness, Vincent says that he was just getting cleaned up. Jules replies, "I used the same fuckin' soap you did and when I got finished the towel didn't look like no goddamn Maxi Pad" (Bender & Tarantino, 1994). The coupling of the words "fuckin', goddamn, and Maxi Pad" captures his disdain and desire to avoid anything that even resembles menstrual blood.

An even greater expression of menstrual avoidance and antipathy by an adult male is heard a few years later in Neil LaBute's *Your Friends and Neighbors*. The scene shows a woman cowering naked in a bathroom while a man outside bangs at the door, paces around the room, and berates her over a menstrual mishap:

> You lied to me, right in my fuckin' person. I'm serious; you are not a nice woman. And who in the fuck just gets her period all of a sudden? It just doesn't happen, and it's happened all over my duvet. You know, you knew that, and you're twisted; you planned this. And I hope to god you have one of those red bio-hazard bags in your purse cause you just bought yourself a set of linens—380 thread count. Bullshit! (He rattles the locked door.) What's the matter? A little sick? Crampy? How about this? Try shoving two aspirins up your crack, and never, ever, fuckin' call me in the morning? Got it? Now I'm goin' down to grab a beer, and I guess some fuckin' 409. Be gone when I get back, OK? (Golin et al., 1998)

The woman has no lines in the scene and she is never seen again. Its sole purpose is to demonstrate the extent of his self-centeredness and exploitive personality. It seems that, according to LaBute, the essence of how men view and treat women can be efficiently reduced to how they react to menstrual encounters.

This misogynist stands in sharp contrast to the male character depicted by another auteur film maker, Mike Leigh, eight years earlier in *Secrets and Lies* (1990) which includes a tender husband bringing a hot water bottle to his wife and trying his best to commiserate. He stands at the foot of the bed and says, "You've drawn the short straw, mate" (Williams & Leigh, 1990). In his case the bewildering experience he is witnessing elicits awe and sympathy in contrast to the fear and rage that the LaBute character expressed. The two men occupy opposite ends of some kind of menstrual sensitivity scale.

On the surface it would not seem that the cad in *Your Friends and Neighbors* would have much in common with the renowned poet T. S. Eliot, but the British biopic *Tom & Viv* portrays Eliot as similarly overwhelmed by a bed-mate's period, in this case that of his wife, Vivienne Heigh-Wood. The film offers up a sad story, one might call it an anti-romance, of how Eliot and his wife (played by Willem Dafoe and Miranda Richardson) became estranged due to her gynecological and emotional problems that made dramatic appearances on their honeymoon. The scene depicts Eliot as being so appalled by his wife's menstrual condition—the sheets are awash in the results of her heavy flow—that he nearly goes into shock. His repulsion is so great that he has to leave her for a walk on the beach where he wades fully clothed in the waves to cleanse himself.

The entire film consists of little more than a series of scenes in which Viv causes one embarrassing emotional fracas after another in desperate attempts to gain the affection of her increasingly alienated, cold and aloof husband. There is no doubt that hormonal imbalance is the cause of her instability as early in the film a close mother-daughter conversation conveys the fact that she is perpetually on the brink of yet another menstrual misstep. The dialogue makes it amply clear as her mother explains that "Viv suffered from women's troubles," asks her "How often is Granny visiting you?" "How often do you get the curse?" and "Have you enough ST's?" [sanitary towels] (Kass et al., 1994). Eventually, Eliot has his wife committed to a mental institution where she spends the rest of her life, even after she enters menopause and, the film makes clear, she has become calm and serene.

Tom & Viv is an extremely rare film in that its entire story line is based on the role of a woman's menstrual cycle on not just *her* life but her husband's as well. One might expect a bio-pic about one of the most famous and influential literary figures of the 20th century to pay more attention to his poetry, but it turns into a virtual case study in male menstruphobia. There is no suggestion that his phobic response to menstrual blood shaped his literary output, but the invitation to speculation is there none-the-less.

Furthermore, it is likely that telling such a story through the life of a famous author and set nearly a century earlier (the couple eloped in 1915) made it possible to explore the taboo and the psychological damage it did to both parties in a more sensitive fashion. And based on the five films considered here, the menstrual closet door was certainly ajar.

The turn of the millennium marked a number of new developments, including those in the realm of cinematic period scenes. Three films in particular warrant attention as they represent shifts that were appearing in the larger menstrual ecology: *The Departed* (2006), directed by Martin Scorsese; *Superbad* (2007), directed by Greg Mottolo, and *Agora* (2009), directed by Alejandro Amenabar.

It is no surprise that Scorsese, given his penchant for stories of macho men in Mafia gangs, police precincts, and socially conservative male dominated institutions, would employ traditional menstrual values as a means of establishing characters and advancing a plot line. Early in *The Departed* as Billy, the Leonardo diCaprio character, is conniving to ingratiate himself into the underworld Boston gang he has been assigned by the police to infiltrate, he is seen standing beside one of the gang members at the bar they hang out in. He orders a cranberry juice and the other man comments, "That's what my wife orders when she's on her period. Are you on your period?" (Grey, King, Nunnari, Pitt, & Scorsese, 2006). Billy pauses just a moment then grabs a glass and smashes it on the man's head. The rudest of all insults, that he could be a woman and, worse yet, be menstruating, is a challenge to his manhood, and the ensuing brawl gives him the opportunity to demonstrate his toughness to the gang's leader and gain acceptance.

Seth, the teenager played by Jonah Hill in *Superbad*, is similarly disturbed by a menstrual connection though his reaction is different. Shortly after he was dancing with a girl who rubbed herself against his leg, he encounters several older guys who ask him about what appears to be a bloodstain on his pants leg. One of the guys rubs his finger on it, holds it up for him to see and asks, "Were you dancing with some chick in there?" It takes several moments for him to realize that there is menstrual blood on him and he begins to gag. He looks around desperately and exclaims, "I'm gonna fuckin' throw up. Someone perioded on my fuckin' leg?" The older guys laugh and call others over to witness the humiliation and even take snapshots of it. They shout to others at the party, "This jerk off's got period blood on his pants," someone says he has a "mangina" and several of the girls offer him a tampon. He pushes his way through the crowd to the basement where he grabs containers of laundry soap and runs out of the house (Apatow & Mottolo, 2007).

Although the man in *The Departed* is older and the setting is earlier and the two movies are of completely different genres, the underlying need for men to distance themselves from any association with menstruation is equally strong. The boy's reaction is played for laughs and the man's is viciously violent, yet the power that menstrual fear has over both of them is striking.

Agora was released a few years later; however, it is set in Roman Egypt nearly 2000 years ago. The director, Alejandro Amenabar, based the film on the historical character Hypatia of Alexandria, a famed philosopher and mathematics professor, and he included a scene that has become part of the lore surrounding this feminist icon. Hypatia (Rachel Weisz) is seen lecturing her class of young men on philosophical and astrological matters. According to legend, one of her students, an arrogant man of privilege, had developed a crush on her and, rather than showing respect for her intellect, expressed his romantic desires. The next day Hypathia brings to the lecture arena a package and places it before him. He opens it to find a pile of her bloody menstrual rags. He is made to understand that he is expressing his base lust, not appreciation for her mind or her spirit. This is a softened version of the encounter. In written accounts she is said to have reached under her robe right in front of the class and pulled out her menstrual rags to humiliate the young man. In the film he leaves the room in disgrace (Bovaira, Augustin, & Amenabar, 2009).

Amenabar has given full credit to the historical character. His way of providing her with agency is to show her turning the menstrual tables upside down by rejecting shame and using the negatives to her advantage. Not only has the shunned suitor been taught a lesson but also all of the other young men in the class have been given a practicum in ancient feminism. Unfortunately, *Agora* did not receive as wide an audience as the others being discussed, but it did broaden the parameters of menstrual elements in feature films. And in a way it approached the topic similar to the technique used in the previous decade's *Tom & Viv* by building it around an actual historical character set in a time that was remote from that of the viewing audience.

As menstruation has steadily become less "unmentionable" across the entire social and media spectrum, films have become more matter-of-fact in their representations. A striking example is found in the 2017 release, *20th Century Women* (Carey & Mills), which makes that very shift the center piece of the most memorable scene in the film by contrasting the views of women of two different generations regarding the permissibility of even mentioning the topic in a social setting. The film is set in 1979 in Santa Barbara, California. The main character, Dorothea (Annette Bening) is a single mother with a son in his mid teens. To make ends meet she takes in boarders including two twenty-something women named Abbie (Greta Gerwig) and Julie (Elle Fanning) as well as a fortyish man named William (Billy Crudup). Faced with the challenges of raising a young boy, she sometimes seeks her boarders' advice on delicate topics.

The big scene takes place at a dinner party. Ten people aged from teens to older adult are sitting around the table; Dorothea, the mother, is in the center smoking a cigarette. Across from her. Abbie is slouched down with her head resting on the table. She tells her son who is sitting next to Abbie to wake her but when he does, she snaps at him, "Stop it, I'm menstruating." Dorothea chides her for her lack of modesty, but Abbie takes the opportunity to give the young boy an impromptu lesson in women's anatomy: "If you ever want to have an adult relationship with a woman, like if you ever want to have sex with a woman's vagina, you need to be comfortable with the fact that the vagina menstruates. And just say menstruation; it's not a big deal" (Carey, et. al. & Mills, 2017).

She proceeds to get the boy to say the word "menstruation" several times with increasing emphasis and then goes around the table directing all the other males to say "menstruation" as well leading up to having the entire group recite the word in unison. Then, William, at the end of the table, takes it one step further speaking to Jamie. He explains, "And sex during menstruation can be very pleasurable for a woman and it can even relieve some of the cramps. And, Jamie, I just want to say never have sex with a woman with just the vagina. You have to have sex with the whole woman" (Carey & Mills, 2017).

Dorothea looks on with disgust at this flagrant violation of the menstrual rules of order. There is a generational divide when it comes to airing menstrual information in front of men and, worse yet, at the dinner table. Though the movie is set in 1979, the values expressed are more reflective of the time of the film's release. Responses to it on social media reflect the change. On the YouTube site the dinner clip has received a lot of attention with over 25,000 hits and dozens of comments. The idea of having William, the handyman and sensitive guy, informing Jamie that having sex during the period might be pleasurable is another nuance. The difference between him and the long list of his cinematic predecessors who found even the thought of menstruation loathsome let alone willingly—even eagerly!—having sex with a menstruating woman is a striking development.

As the preceding discussion demonstrates, menstruation in film has undergone a steady evolution. Looking back upon the variety of menstrual details that have shown up in feature films it is possible to offer a few tentative conclusions. The earliest (other than when mention of the cessation of menstruation was used as a way of introducing a pregnancy) were drawn from novels, e.g., *Carrie* and *To Sir, with Love*. I suggest that it was easier to justify including menstrual material, and any other potentially objectionable topic, in a mainstream feature film if it was based on an adaptation of a novel. After all, books are a far more "respectable" art form and a book-based film may be more resistant to the censor's scissors. Furthermore, these two books had already passed muster and had even been accepted for adolescent reading lists so the plot lines held little surprise or shock value. Meanwhile, as audiences and consumers of all media have become more accepting of images and subject matter that would have been forbidden by custom, policy or legislation in earlier decades, there are still restrictions in place. While blood flows freely on the screen if it is the result or injuries sustained in war, crime, disease or other means of mayhem, the appearance of menstrual blood is still rare. Quick glimpses of a stained sheet or back of a skirt with a red spot are more common than previously, but the level of acceptance is drastically different. It remains to be seen if the ongoing shifts in menstrual acceptance will find expression in even greater explicitness in feature films

Film and Television References

Apatow, J. (Producer), & Mottola, G. (Director). (2007). *Superbad* [Motion Picture]. United States: Columbia Pictures.

Bender, L. (Producer), & Tarantino, Q. (Director). (1994). *Pulp Fiction* [Motion Picture]. United States: Miramax.

Bovaira, F., Augustin, A. (Producers), & Amenabar, A. (Director). (2009). *Agora* [Motion Picture]. Spain: Focus Features.

Brabourne, J. (Producer), & Zeffirelli, F. (Director). (1968). *Romeo and Juliet* [Motion Picture]. United Kingdom: BHE Films.

Brower, M. (Producer), & Altman, R. (Director). (1971). *McCabe & Mrs. Miller* [Motion Picture]. United States: David Foster Productions.

Carey, A., Ellison, M., Henley, Y. (Producers), & Mills, M. (Director). (2016). *20th Century Women* [Motion Picture]. United States: Annapurna Pictures.

Carr, A. (Producer), & Kleiser, R. (Director). (1978). *Grease* [Motion Picture]. United States: Paramount Pictures.

Castle, W. (Producer), & Polanksi, R. (Director). (1968). *Rosemary's Baby* [Motion Picture]. United States: William Castle Productions.

Chartoff, R. (Producer), & Pollack, S. (1969). *They Shoot Horses, Don't They?* [Motion Picture]. United States: Palomar Pictures.

Clavell, J. (Producer & Director). (1967). *To Sir, with Love* [Motion Picture]. United States: Columbia Pictures.

Dougherty, M. (Producer), & Ritchie, M. (1975). *Smile* [Motion Picture]. United States: David V. Picker Productions.

Fox, F. (Creator). (1952). *My Little Margie* [Television Series]. Culver City, CA: NBC.

Gilbert, R. (Producer), & Perry, F. (Director). (1970). *Diary of a Mad Housewife* [Motion Picture]. United States: Frank Perry Films Inc.

Goldstone, J. (Producer), & Gilliam T., Jones, T. (Directors). (1983). *Monty Python's The Meaning of Life* [Motion Picture]. United Kingdom: Celandine Films, Universal Pictures.

Golin, S., Patric, J. (Producers), & LaBute, N. (Director). (1998) *Your Friends and Neighbors* [Motion Picture]. United States: PolyGram Filmed Entertainment.

Grey, B., King, G., Nunnari, G., Pitt, B. (Producers), & Scorsese, M. (Director). (2006). *The Departed* [Motion Picture]. United States: Warner Bros.

Green, H. (Producer), & Hughes, J. (Director). (1984). *Sixteen Candles* [Motion Picture] United States: Universal Pictures.

Hitchcock, A. (Producer & Director). (1960). *Psycho* [Motion Picture]. United States: Shamley Productions.

James, E. (Creator). (1954). *Father Knows Best* [Television Series]. Burbank, CA: NBC.

Jewison, N. (Producer & Director). (1985). *Agnes of God* [Motion Picture]. United States: Columbia Pictures Corporation.

Joffe, C. (Producer), & Allen, W. (Director). (1977). *Annie Hall* [Motion Picture]. United States: Jack Rollins & Charles H. Joffe Productions.

Kass, H., Samuelson, M., Samuelson, P. (Producers), & Gilbert, B. (Director). (1994). *Tom & Viv* [Motion Picture]. United Kingdom: Miramax.

Kleiser, R. (Producer & Director). (1980). *Blue Lagoon* [Motion Picture]. United States: Columbia Pictures Corporation.

Lewis, E. (Producer), & Frankenheimer, J. (Director). (1968). *The Fixer* [Motion Picture]. United Kingdom: Metro-Goldwyn-Mayer.

Lovell, D. (Producer), & Zeffirelli, F. (Director). (1981). *Endless Love* [Motion Picture]. United States: PolyGram Filmed Entertainment.

Mazursky, P. (Producer & Director). (1978). *An Unmarried Woman* [Motion Picture]. United States: Twentieth Century Fox.

Monash, P. (Producter), & De Palma, P. (Director). (1976). *Carrie* [Motion Picture]. United States: Red Bank Films.

Monash, P. (Producer), & Shea, K. (Director). (1999). *The Rage: Carrie 2* [Motion Picture]. United States: United Artists, Red Bank Films.

Rudin, S. (Producer), & Heckerling, A. (Director). (1995). *Clueless* [Motion Picture]. United States: Paramount Pictures.

Stigwood, R. (Producer), & Badham, J. (Director). (1977). *Saturday Night Fever* [Motion Picture]. United States: Robert Stigwood Organization.

Thalberg, I. (Producer), & Cukor, G. (Director). (1936). *Romeo and Juliet.* [Motion Picture]. United States: Metro-Goldwyn-Mayer Studios.

Vachon, C., Van Sant, G., Woods, C. (Producers), & Clark, L. (Director). (1995). *Kids* [Motion Picture]. United States: Independent Pictures.

Wasserstein, W. (Writer). (1979). *Uncommon Women...and Others* [Television Series]. Hartford, CT: Connecticut Public Television.

Williams, S. (Producer), & Leigh, M. (Director). (1996). *Secrets and Lies.* [Motion Picture]. United States: Channel Four Films.

Print References

Braithwait, E. R. (1959). *To sir, with love*. London: Bodley Head.

Delaney, J., Lupton, M. J., & Toth, E. (1976). *The curse: A cultural history of menstruation*. Chicago, IL: University of Illinois Press.

King, S. (1974). *Carrie*. New York, NY: Doubleday.

Spencer, S. (1979). *Endless love*. New York, NY: Harper Collins.

CHAPTER SEVEN

Selling the Product

Men in Menstrual Marketing

Given that men do not use menstrual pads and tampons it might seem unlikely for them to appear in advertisements for such products. However, the fact that "sex appeal" is one of the staples of advertising appeal for anything, men are often present though usually in subtle and indirect ways. After all, ads for men's shaving products, deodorants, clothing and nearly every other male focused sales pitch commonly includes women who are attracted to the man because he uses the item on sale. However, due to the delicacy and deeply ingrained discretion regarding menstruation, male presence in menstrual product advertising has, until recently, tended to be more implicit than actual.

I have previously documented the history of male presence in menstrual product ads with particular attention to the emphasis on modesty and secrecy, the selling point being a guaranteed that men would never be able to discern that the users of Kotex or Tampax or Modess or Fibs were actually menstruating. Other products, douches such as Lysol and Zonite, promised to preserve marital bliss if women purged themselves of the "offensive odor" associated with menstruation that could alienate husbands and drive them out to the house. That essay, published in the journal *Women & Health* in 2007 traced the history from 1920 through 1949 with focus on the significant changes brought about as a result of World War II and the increased presence of women in factories as well as their role in supporting men in the military (Linton, 2007). This history has also been well documented by Kissling (2006), Vostal (2008), and others. For readers interested in viewing the advertisements cited in the earlier study as well as a wide variety of others from the same era, the best archive of such material is located at the Duke University site, AdAccess.

The following discussion picks up where the earlier essay concluded. The rise of television's ubiquitous presence brought new challenges and opportunities to menstrual product advertising efforts.

Television Gets Into the (Menstrual) Act

In the midst of all of the adjustments being made in the hard-won era of peace and prosperity following the war and the shifts to a more conservative political and social climate expressed in the election of Dwight Eisenhower, a "manly" war hero, as President, a revolutionary technological phenomenon occurred, the introduction of a television set into virtually every home in the country.

In addition to the changes and reversals instigated by the post-war demand that women return to traditional roles, the arrival of television on the entertainment and communication landscape had far reaching effects. In its early days the number of channels the average home had access to was commonly as few as three or four, and in some areas even fewer. Unlike magazines which could be highly specialized and marketed to targeted audiences—separate titles for men, women, boys, girls, and focused interests as well—early television was a universal medium and all of its content had to be deemed "acceptable for family viewing." The slight exception to this rule was to identify certain times of the day as more suited for market segments. The presumption that women were staying at home, men were at work, and children were at school led to the view that the hours between 9:00 am and 4:00 pm were women's viewing hours and the programming of soap operas and other content thought to appeal to "the housewife" dominated the schedule. The evening hours of 6:00 pm to 10:00 pm—prime time—was to be filled with drama, situation comedies, variety shows and other genres appealing to shared family viewing.

Advertisers jumped at the opportunity to pitch products to the captive audiences who were devoted to their favorite programs and who dutifully stayed tuned during the frequent commercial interruptions (there were no remote control channel changers). Many corporations even sponsored and produced entire series so they would have complete access to viewers for the full length of the hour-long program. Naturally the manufacturers of menstrual products wanted to have access to their targeted consumers; however, from its earliest days, content regulation (or censorship) was deemed necessary in the television industry. Even the most covert mention of anything having to do with the "private parts" of women's bodies had to be approached with the utmost discretion.

In 1951 the National Association of Broadcasters, the industry group established in 1922 to deal with government regulation and allocation of broadcast frequencies and licenses, adopted a strict "code" that was rigorously applied to all programming and advertising, including what products could and could not be offered. For instance, ads for hard liquor were not permitted but ads for beer and wine were. The content of the code provides clear insights into a full range of American social attitudes regarding politics, religion, entertainment, social and gender roles, child rearing and a host of other topics, including the proper place of menstruation. Consider the following statement from the 1959, fifth edition of the NAB Code. The language may seem coy or even evasive but network and station executives as well as advertising agencies and product manufacturers were well aware of its meaning:

> The advertising of intimately personal products which are generally regarded as unsuitable conversational topics in mixed social groups is not acceptable. (Anon, 1959, p. 6)

The NAB code continued to be the guiding document for television content until 1982 when a U.S. District Court Judge ruled that the requirements stated in the document violated the Sherman Anti-Trust Act. The Association quickly accepted the ruling and abandoned the code without appealing the decision, leaving the task of policing what went on the air up to networks and local stations (Mayer, 1982).

This did not mean that there was suddenly a flood of explicit programming and previously forbidden products being offered. Broadcasters were still sensitive to their audience's tastes and prejudices and continued to avoid anything that might offend. Networks and stations adopted "Standards and Practices" policies and the portions of those documents pertaining to menstrual products are titled, "Personal Products Advertising Guidelines." Advertisers and programmers were expected to be familiar with these doctrines and craft their material accordingly. Menstrual products continued to be viewed cautiously. Euphemisms were common; however, the term "personal products" was understood to refer to anything having to do with menstruation, incontinence and other "delicate" topics. In order to demonstrate how menstrual product acceptance slowly developed, consider the terminology that was employed in 2003 at the NBC and ABC networks (R. Weiner, personal communication, July 7, 2003):

NBC PERSONAL PRODUCTS—2003
Catamenial Devices and Panty Shields

1. Straight-forward statements of grooming, freshness and femininity, absorbency, duration of efficacy, cleanliness, etc., are acceptable.
2. Use of mixed social situations is limited to incidental appearances.

ABC PERSONAL PRODUCTS—2003
The ABC Personal Products Guidelines apply to all products advertised as personal products: catamenial devices, panty shields, douche products, pregnancy test kits, personal care and grooming products, personal non-prescription medications, undergarments, and incontinence products.

Product Categories
A. Catamenial Devices, Panty Shields, Douche Products
1. Personal products may be depicted provided the execution is restrained and in good taste....
2. The use of either children or mixed social situations in advertising is acceptable when incidental and unrelated to the product.
3. These products may not be promoted for reasons of health.

For contrast, here are the guidelines that were in effect in 2017 at the NBC and ABC networks:

NBC PERSONAL PRODUCTS—2017
Products and services of a personal nature including, but not limited to, feminine hygiene products, personal lubricants, contraceptives, incontinence products and other products that require sensitivity in presentation should be presented in a tasteful manner and will be accepted on a case-by-case basis. Scheduling restrictions may apply. (NBC, 2017, p. 27)

ABC PERSONAL CARE PRODUCTS—2017
Personal care products (such as deodorants, feminine hygiene products, undergarments, and incontinence products) should be presented with utmost care and sensitivity. All copy and visuals must be appropriate and not overly graphic. ABC will consider daypart and program audience composition when scheduling personal product advertising. (ABC, 2017, p. 49)

The most striking thing about the older phrasing is use of the unfamiliar word "catamenial," a term derived form the Greek word, *katamenios*, that means "monthly" and that is used in medical contexts. The use of such arcane language to describe something as common as the menstrual cycle dramatically reveals how intent the regulators were on keeping the topic at a distance. One means of identifying the level of social discomfort associated with any topic is to consider how evasive or euphemistic the language is surrounding the topic. "Making love" often has little to do with love, and "passing away" hardly captures the impact of the matter being described. By this measure "menstruation" must rank among the very most delicate topics imaginable, at least if measured by the plethora of expressions used to allude to it such as "catamenial." So it is a sign of greater acceptance that the word was abandoned (though only relatively recently) in favor of "feminine hygiene products." However, the persistence of the word "hygiene" reinforces the notion that there is something unhealthy or dirty about menses and the grouping of such products in the same sentence as products for "incontinence" reinforces an unfortunate association.

Television Starts to Open the Menstrual Closet

As the guardians and regulators of taste and acceptability continued to struggle with what could pass muster with the TV audience, the creators of ads for menstrual products pushed the boundaries of acceptability. One of the chief ways that they did so was to violate the old rule against having any male presence in settings where menstrual products are mentioned. To illustrate just how far things have come since the days of catamenial evasion, consider two examples of ads for Tampax products that were aired during the 2003–2004 programming season. Though in the new generation of ads men were in fact quite present, they were often just as much in the dark about menstruation as if they weren't there. To some extent, the old values of secrecy and shame were maintained but with a sense of humor that attempted to move away from shame in the direction of privacy and discretion. The underlying idea was, "We girls have some secrets that guys don't understand and aren't we clever in how we manage them."

A 2004 Tampax Pearl TV spot titled "Boat Leak" opens on a wide shot of a small row boat on a lake. A young man and woman, probably in their early to mid 20's, face each other in the boat. A large white heron flies by in the background. The male is ecstatically praising the beauty of the setting when the woman points out that there is a leak in the boat. The fourth shot is a close up of the floor of the boat where we see the woman's sandaled feet (the straps of her sandals are covered with rows of pearls) and between them an oval shaped hole from which a small spurt of water gushes upward. If one freezes the frame or watches it repeatedly, it becomes clear that the hole is vaginal in shape and that the wood splinters have the appearance of dark pubic hair at the edges. Its placement between her feet invites association with her vagina and the spurt suggests either urine or heavy menstrual flow. The young man says, "I can handle this," and turns away, presumably to get something to bail with or a plug for the hole. While his back is turned, the woman reaches into her bag and pulls out a full box of Tampax Pearl tampons. She quickly unwraps one and reaches down to insert it into the hole in the boat. Though we see the tampon in her hand, we do not see the actual insertion. During this action a female voice-over announcer states, "For protection against unexpected leaks, you need Tampax Pearl because Pearl expands quickly and comfortably." The visual for the second half of this speech is a graphic that demonstrates how the tampon expands when wet. Of course, the demonstration uses blue fluid. Next, the man turns back, glances down and discovers that the woman has solved the problem. The tampon is in place with the string dangling over it. The flow has ceased. The final shot returns to the opening image with the couple leaning toward each other as their romantic date on the lake proceeds, saved by the ingenious use of the Pearl tampon. As the shot fades, the product slogan is superimposed across the scene: "The one, the only, Tampax Pearl."

The Pearl ad is both old fashioned and modern at the same time. It reflects the values of the early TV sit-coms such as *The Honeymooners* or *Father Knows Best* in which women seem to be retiring yet are really the problem solvers. The woman's management of the tampon solution to the boat leak is done quickly and efficiently behind the turned back of her companion and it is not clear if the man realizes exactly how she has solved the problem since he is never facing her when she handles the tampon. And her demeanor is sufficiently shy so that it is not clear if she will explain to him how she saved the day. And it seems unlikely that he will ask. However, it is clear that the continuation of the romantic day on the lake is saved by her having the Pearl tampon handy; and, by extension, the larger message is that use of this product will allow anyone's love life to continue without inter- ruption even though one may be "leaking." The final shot has the man resting his hand on the phallic shaped handle of the oars as they resume their appreciation of nature and each other (Tampax Pearl, 2004).

An ad for another Tampax product, Compak, a tampon with "a discrete plastic applicator," appeared in 2003. It is set in a school classroom, probably tenth or eleventh grade. During its 30 seconds of screen time it squeezes in 17 shots and a full blown dramatic confrontation complete with several characters, an inciting incident, building tension, an amusing resolution, and even an anticlimax, not to mention a pitch for the product. Here's the story:

A girl passes a note across the aisle to her girl friend who reads it, nods, reaches into her purse and hands back a small item. The teacher, a bald, middle-aged man sitting behind his desk at the front of the room says loudly, "Miss McGee, will you bring that to the front please." The students mutter an "oh, oh" kind of sound as the student hands the teacher a small, plastic wrapped object resembling a packaged candy. In a close up shot the teacher holds it up in front of his face and says, "Well, I hope you brought enough for everyone." The girl, looking quizzical but not upset, responds, "Enough for the girls." The last shot in the drama shows several boys in an adjacent row looking confused as though they don't get what the girls are giggling about. A woman's narrator voice cuts in stating, "Tampax Compak is so discrete only you'll know it's a tampon," and a screen shot shows the tampon out of its wrapper. The ad closes with the announcer stating, "Small size, big protection. The one, the only, Tampax Compak" (Tampax Conpak, 2003).

When a film moves along as quickly as this one with no single shot held on screen longer than a few seconds, the audience has little opportunity to examine the subtleties of shot composition, small details within the shots or other elements that the writers and directors selected with great care. Furthermore, the low level of attention given ads has always been a challenge to advertisers, and this problem has only increased due to the presence of remote control devices that allow audiences to cut away to other channels or to mute the ads. Advertisers have two solutions to these problems. One has been to show the same ads over and over again, sometimes even two or more times within a single advertising cluster, and the other has been to make the ads more entertaining by the introduction of humor, catchier music, engaging story lines and over-all higher production values. What is especially daring about the Tampax Pearl ad is that it manages to place vivid symbolic images of female genitals and heavy menstrual flow within the context of a romantic relationship story played out in a bucolic setting. In both ads gender relationships are the basis of the drama and the way the women use their tampons is such that they appear to be superior in some way to the clueless men they are dealing with. The young man in the boat who thought he was going to plug the hole and save the day is seen as less inventive and able than the woman with her handy tampon. Viewers are left wondering what other purposes she might find for this handy device—a sort of Swiss Army Tampon!

In the classroom setting the girl is poised and sure of herself in the face of the male teacher who becomes a foil for her joke. The audience is left to imagine what will happen next when the teacher realizes that he is waving around a girl's tampon which was about to be used for its intended purpose. It is he, not the girl, who is going to be embarrassed by this transaction, and the confusion and ignorance on the faces of the boys in the room further enhances her mastery of the situation. None-the-less, the voice over commentary reinforces the importance of secrecy, or at least discretion, "Only you'll know it's a tampon." The two ads managed to defy the conservative impulse against male presence while skirting the edges of taste and propriety. In one sense the assumption of shame, or at least secrecy, is maintained while the young women in the ads are depicted as clever and resourceful in their management of the appurtenances of their periods.

Menstrual Media Case Studies

Over time it has become increasingly difficult to pin down the relationship between the role of advertising in reinforcing social values versus challenging values in the interest of selling a product or service. There are several reasons for this. First, the ephemeral nature of advertising with new marketing campaigns for a given product emerging frequently makes it hard to chart historical developments. Second, competition among different manufacturers of products with little or no differences between the products themselves leads to campaigns that are often based on style or celebrity presence or some other unrelated element. Third, there are no readily accessible archives or libraries that collect and index advertising. There is no advertising equivalent of the IMDB site that provides thorough information on film production right down to budget details. Fourth, again unlike movies, advertising campaigns are not readily transported from country to country. Advertisers are sensitive to local customs and craft their message accordingly which can mean that an ad that is successful in one setting may be offensive in another. Fifth, though advertisers tend to create campaign strategies that can apply to both print and televising, the inherent differences in the two media can result in significant nuances. Magazine appeal tends to be much more targeted so that the pitch to the narrowly defined readership of *Cosmopolitan* magazine, for instance, will be more focused than a TV ad for the same product on a network TV show.

As a result of these unique characteristics the following discussion will take the shape of a set of case studies of campaigns and individual examples, all of which (with a few exceptions) address the central theme of this book: what are the roles men have been assigned in shaping the message; how do menstrual transactions influence the marketing of menstrual products?

Period Sex

While television advertising has made cautious strides in opening up the story lines in skits and dramatizations to include male presence, it has (so far) drawn the line at any overt suggestion that couples might actually have sexual relations while the woman had her period. Magazine ads are under no such restrictions as several full page ads for Instead Softcup, a disposable alternative to pads and tampons, makes clear. There is no evasiveness in the copy which states, "… you can have mess-free sex, even when you have your period." The campaign used two sexually provocative photo illustrations. One shows a young couple kissing and holding hands seen through a narrow opening in a pair of thick curtains. They are back-lit by a window and might even be thought to be hiding behind the drapes.

The ad is a semiotician's delight. Everything surrounding the couple reads "old fashioned." The drapes are dark and tattered; a mantel on the left has a gilded picture frame, floral wall paper and the edge of a deer's antlers mounted high on the wall; the bottom of the picture fades into darkness. However, at the bottom edge is a box of the Softcup product, angled in such a way as to appear to be emerging from the dark room. The large print imposed on the dark curtains states, "Do everything you would if you didn't have your period. We're not just talking about swimming."

The text at the bottom drives home the notion that this is a new product for a new generation that is less squeamish about sex during menstruation. The emphasis is on the idea that the cup will contain the menstrual flow so that you can go about your life just as though you didn't even have a period. And, ironically, that appeal turns the ad into a reaffirmation of the anti-period sex stereotype. Though posing as a hip new product to appeal to young women who presumably are not hampered by antiquated notions of when in the cycle it is OK to have sex, the ad implies that, just like the long tradition in pad and tampon ads, you can go about your life as though you did not have a period. In other words, it's another appeal to "keep him from knowing."

Another ad in the series takes the message even further. The full-page photo has a voyeuristic quality as we gaze through an open door into a bedroom. Only the lower portion of the bed is visible so that a couple's naked legs can be seen. The image is made particularly titillating by the fact that the woman has kept on her somewhat spiky heeled shoes suggesting urgency as well as a hint of kinkiness. What's more, the woman is on top, an image of assertiveness and power that is reflected in the text at the bottom, "So now your period can't stop you from indulging in all your favorite activities, whatever they may be." Furthermore, the "woman superior" position (as it used to be called in sex manuals) also implies that the cup is so effective that there's no danger of having your blood stream out onto your partner, even when you're straddling him.

Since these ads appeared in 2011 the promotional efforts have taken another turn, including an amusing poke at the competition with the tag line, "More freedom during your period—no strings attached." Nonetheless, there is still the prevailing sense that menstrual management should remain a matter that men are to be spared knowledge of.

Menstrual Marketing Down Under

Although menstruation is a universal phenomenon that happens to nearly all women everywhere in the world, it would be a mistake to assume that is viewed the same universally. Even countries with a common language and similar colonial histories and economic systems can vary in how they perceive acceptable menstrual marketing. Two TV ads from Australia illustrate the point. Neither is likely to have ever been acceptable for screening on broadcast television in most other English-speaking countries during the time they ran in their homeland. One takes a gentle swipe at some of the stereotypes regarding women's menstrual bonding practices and the other takes risks with colloquial genital slang.

The first, an ad for Cottons tampons titled "Sympathy Pains," was produced in 2001 and went on to win industry awards for the Young & Rubicam Agency in Melbourne. It features four actors, all of them men.

The opening shot is a wide view of a city construction site on what looks like a traffic island. The sounds of traffic and a pneumatic drill are heard. The second shot closes in on a young, stringy haired man operating the drill who stops and mutters, "I don't think I can do this much longer." The foreman, a big-bellied older fellow with a walrus mustache growls, "What the hell is it now!?"

The young worker sheepishly says, "I've got cramps. I've got my period."

Suddenly concerned, the foreman replies, "Oh, OK, All right, better relax then. Sit down for a moment. Big breaths... You know, I always use a hot water bottle."

A work mate calls from the side, "Want a herbal tea, Pat?"

"No, no, no, I'm all right."

The boss continues, "Put it across the tummy. Just relaxes, takes the pain out. It's brilliant. It's really good."

Another worker chimes in, "My Dad did the same thing."

"It's great..." continues the boss.

The young man then mutters that's he's OK and resumes his work with the drill but the boss assures him, "If it gets too much again, we'll put someone else on it." The scene fades to a black screen with the title, "IF ONLY," followed by shot of the product, a box of Cottons tampons. There is no voice over and the product name is on screen for a few brief seconds (Cottons, 2001).

This entertaining ad efficiently captures details associated with women's tribal lore: conversations and practices known to and shared orally by women across ages and classes but about which men are commonly kept in the dark. The bonding the men express, the sharing of lore (hot water bottles, "My Dad did the same thing," herbal tea), the caring for one another, are all common expressions of women's experience that are usually kept within the "tribe." The fact that the director of the piece and the two producers were women (Vikki Blanche, Helene Nicole and Leanne Tonkes) subverts potential charges that the ad is hostile to women. The ad suggests a turning point may have been reached, at least in Australia, a gradual shift in the menstrual ecology, the ways men and women, both individually and collectively, conduct their menstrual encounters. Notions of secrecy, whether to expose or withhold information thought to belong exclusively to one tribe or a subset of a tribe, are opened and found amusing.

On the surface, the second item, a 2008 ad for U by Kotex appears to be nothing other than a peppy 30 second jaunt featuring a young woman going about a variety of pleasant activities with her pet. She strolls down the street with it in her arms; they visit a hair salon where it sits on a pile of magazines beneath a dryer next to her; they get their nails painted together; they lie on the beach on adjacent towels where two handsome men stop to gaze at them appreciatively; at a restaurant she gives her pet to a present wrapped in a bow. The noteworthy—and controversial—thing about the spot is that her pet is a large brown beaver, its flat tail and sharp front teeth visible in most of the shots. Yes, the woman is treating her beaver well, as the voice over at the closing shot of the gift, a box of Kotex tampons, says, "You've only got one, so for the ultimate care—down there—make it U" (Kotex, 2008).

The closing line and picture of the beaver opening the box have strong shock value. The viewer is required to flash back through the story and realize that the pet she seems to have with her at all times and takes such loving care of is meant to stand for her genitals. And repeated viewings make the production even richer. There are many women extras in the background of the salon, the street and the beach, and closer examination discovers that every one of them is also lugging a beaver around with her. Better yet, the hair color of each woman's beaver matches the hair color of the woman who is carrying it. Of course! But the most daring visual element is the beach scene where two men stop to smile and stare admiringly at her and her beaver sprawling on the sand. No wonder the ad stirred controversy.

Immediately upon its initial screening television stations received complaints about the implication that a slang word for genitals was being used though the only words spoken in the ad was the closing tag line. Product representatives responded that the use of "beaver" as a playful name for vagina was the result of research into the terms women use to refer to their genitals. They claimed that most women in their target audience (18 to 24) had euphemisms or "pet names" for their genitals, including 181 different terms. "Beaver" was the 11th-most common (Cummings & Howden, 2008).

Despite the amount of attention the ad received and claims that sales and brand exposure had increased due to the attention it garnered, the company decided not to use the new mascot on TV again but it did continue to show up in social media marketing. And there was some question as to whether the beaver was male or female; there were assurances made that the beaver was indeed female (Hicks, 2012).

Conclusion

The institution of advertising is both a mechanism for maintaining the status quo and at the same time an instrument of change. It is both ephemeral and substantial. Its immensity and complexity make it impossible to fully archive its manifestations. Any attempt to identify exhaustively its influence is bound to come up short. However, it is hoped that the aspects touched upon in the preceding paragraphs and the examples offered for examination have provided both models for further exploration and perspectives on how the marketing of menstrual products demonstrates how men and women share in the maintenance and the modification of the complex constellation of menstrual transactions.

References to Television Ads

Cottons. (2001). Sympathy Pains. Retrieved November 5, 2018 from https://www.youtube.com/watch?v=gfisTUx-DKI

Kotex. (2008). Beaver. Retrieved November 5, 2018 from https://www.youtube.com/watch?v=RkkTeAP8d5o

Tampax Compak. (2003). Classroom. Retrieved November 5, 2018 from https://www.youtube.com/watch?v=ZUoXGr26_Rs

Tampax Pearl. (2004). Boat Leak. Retrieved November 5, 2018 from https://www.youtube.com/watch?v=2tufXp1Of6g

References

ABC. (2017). ABC Television network advertising standards and guidelines. Retrieved November 5, 2018 from https://abcallaccess.com/app/uploads/2016/01/2014-Advertising-Guidelines-.pdf

Anon. (1959). The television code of the National Association of Broadcasters. Retrieved November 5, 2018 from http://www.tv-signoffs.com/1959_NAB_Television_Code.pdf

Cummings, I., & Howden, S. (2008, March 10). Kotex tampons' beaver advertisement denounced. *The Daily Telegraph*. Retrieved July 12, 2018 from https://www.dailytelegraph.com.au/ kotex-tampons-beaver-advertisment-denounced/news-story/d0bcd3054d268dad5d4cfe c2497790e0?sv=bb829d47fb2adc71db5ded4a1eb36732

Hicks, R. (2012, April 3). U by Kotex marketer: The beaver won't go on TV because it was spoiling our messaging. *Mumbrella*. Retrieved July 12, 2018 from https://mumbrella. com.au/u-by-kotex-marketer-the-beaver-wont-go-on-tv-because-it-was-spoiling-our-messaging-83120

Kissling, L. (2006). *Capitalizing on the curse: The business of menstruation*. Boulder, CO: Lynne Rienner.

Linton, D. (2007). Men in menstrual product advertising: 1920–1949. *Women & Health, 46*(1), 99–114.

Mayer, C. (1982, March 11). NAB to halt enforcement of ad code. *Washington Post*. Retrieved July 12, 2018 from https://www.washingtonpost.com/archive/business/1982/03/11/nab-to-halt-enforcement-of-ad-code/956e5098-8594-4018-85e2-f3762e416129/?noredi rect=on&utm_term=.33847aa212de

NBC (2017). NBCUniversal advertising standards. Retrieved November 5, 2018 from https://www.nbcuadstandards.com/files/NBC_Network_Advertising_Guidelines. pdf;jsessionid=8DD5A6B39CECA1D7B160171F4C5F298E

Vostal, S (2008). *Under wraps: A history of menstrual hygiene technology*. New York, NY: Lexington Books.

CHAPTER EIGHT

Making Menstrual Music

Singing the Menstrual Blues

An examination of music history yields few mentions of menstruation. Whether it be classical opera, folk music or the popular standards of Broadway, menstruation was not in the song book. Neither Frank Sinatra nor Peggy Lee sang of the period (unless one thinks that the latter's "Fever" had something to do with hot flashes). However, just as the barriers have come down in the realm of film, television, literature, and casual conversation, modern audiences bandy around the initials PMS and even sing about it. At the time of this writing a search of "PMS Blues" on the iTunes app found 17 separate songs with that title. More broadly, a search of the term "pms" yielded 100 titles, though 62 of them are for a band called "P.M.S.," few of whose songs have anything to do with menstruation. A search for "menstruation" produced 88 hits. Many of these are duplicates indicating that the song appeared on more than one album and some are references to bands that had the word in their name such as Menstruation Monsters but did not include specific menstrual references in the lyrics. Furthermore, many of the selections are instrumentals which invites the question: what about an instrumental piece of music would suggest that it be titled with a reference to menstruation? As it turns out the answer is that many of the pieces are either wild punk or heavy metal pieces with shrieking guitars engaged in long shredding solos. And these lists do not include the numerous songs that include passing mention of a menstrual detail as in Janet

Jackson's "Feedback" when she describes her appeal as, "My swag is serious. I'm heavy like a first day period" (Daniels, Emile, Jerkins, & Yasin, 2007).

Not every mention of blood and women in the same line is meant to be menstrual. As unlikely as it seems, Alice Cooper has claimed that "Only Women Bleed" (Cooper & Wagner, 1975) is meant to depict the pain of a woman in an abusive relationship, not that he was singing about the menstrual cycle. In fact, in an attempt to disassociate the song from the menstrual connection, the official title was later changed to "Only Women."

In those songs that are intended to make a point about menstrual transactions, it is interesting to note how men and women differ in perception. Of the 17 songs listed in the iTunes catalog under PMS Blues, eight are written and/or voiced by women, and nine are identified as reflecting the male experience. And in every case a portion of the lyrics pertain to how the presence of menstruation impacts the relationship the menstruator has with others, notably men. However, in the case of songs by women, there is also usually an emphasis on topics such as the individual's physical discomfort and other personal matters while in the men's songs the focus is solely on how the woman's period affects his feelings, fears, desires, and behavior.

The longest and most robust woman's song in the P.M.S. Blues list is a 5 and a half minute recording of a live performance by the country music star Dolly Parton. Departing from the traditional "always love your man" trope, Parton sets out on a roaring rant about how miserable her menstrual cycle is. But, rather than coming off as a plea for pity, she sounds like a defiant warrior. And the audience loves it! The whooping and cheering heard from women's voices in the crowd serve as a massive Amen Choir endorsing her sentiments while rejoicing in the audacity of bringing the topic out in the open before her adoring fans and defying the prohibition against public mention of "women's troubles." The song opens with a nearly sacrilegious attack on the source of all menstrual blues:

Eve you wicked woman
You done put your curse on me
Why didn't you just leave that apple hangin' in the tree? (Parton, 1994)

It proceeds from there through a catalog of all the bad feelings and behavior she has exhibited due to her period, even how it makes her feel about herself. At times there is an apologetic tone as when she identifies the victims of her rage; men.

Returning to the revivalist, evangelical style of the opening of the song, she invites the audience to join her in testifying to the truth of her sermon with a series of three "Can I get a witness?!" calls to the crowd, first to the women, who scream their agreement, then to the men who also shout their endorsement of the premise that women are irrational crazies during their periods, and finally even the children in the audience are invited to witness with the invitation, "Do you wanna talk about the mean old devil mamma of yours?" Having firmly established the idea that PMS makes being a woman a hellish condition, she goes one step further by confessing that sometimes her PMS even made her wish she were a man. In the middle of the song, she points out that this piece could only have been written by a woman. The fact that Dolly Parton has built her career in part on embodying in style, appearance, and song choices the very essence of traditional female attributes within the country music tradition makes this song all the more noteworthy, not to mention that despite the fact that she was born in 1946 and it was not recorded until 1994 she has continued to perform it well past the time she has most likely ceased menstruating. Her elevated status has made it possible for her to flaunt the period in ways that a younger, less established woman would find a risky enterprise.

Other women singers who have addressed the impact of pre-menstrual syndrome in their lives have been somewhat less demonstrative and the collective impact provides some interesting nuances.

American Gypsy's "P.M.S. Blues" (Anon., 2003) story is presented on an album titled *Let me be … free* that features a cover photo of a young "biker chic" with a long braid straddling a Harley-Davidson motorcycle. The song opens with the line

How many women with PMS does it take to change a light bulb?
It takes one…

The song proceeds to grumble about how no one does anything correctly, including taking out the garbage or changing a light bulb. Though those inept individuals who make her life miserable are not identified as men, the implication is clear. Unlike most of the other songs that include lists of the many rude and nasty feelings and behaviors the singer engages in, instead this one includes a long list of "treatments" such as ice cream, candy, vodka, and a variety of drugs.

Two different treatments of another song titled "P.M.S. Blues" are offered by Christiane Noll (Noll, 2014) and a duo called Kathy & Shanti (Budway, 2000). The song is essentially a mix of lamentation and apology:

It happens every month that I feel like I'm losing my mind
I try to do something but I only end up wastin' my time.

The woman described in these lyrics is, by her own accounting, terrifying. She can barely tolerate herself and gives fair warning to anyone who happens to be in her proximity that they should expect to be treated badly. The song ends with the singer making a prolonged shriek that captures both her misery and her scariness. She sees herself as both a wreck—and a wrecker.

Another release included in the P.M.S. Blues list conflates two different menstrual concerns. Though Cherry & the Violators (Anon., 2007) sing of menstrual mood swings, the opening line identifies a different concern:

Hey, Auntie, why don't you visit me today?
Well I looked it up on my calendar and this time you're really runnin' late.

Although she does mention the fact that her mother told her not to come home until her mood has settled down, it's not the "monthly miseries" she's concerned about. Her boyfriend has grasped the problem clearly: he left to buy cigarettes a week ago and never came back. This song manages to provide a "two for the price of one" look at menstrual concerns: PMS discomforts as well as *not* getting one's period and the worry about having an unintended pregnancy.

Capturing the confessional tone that characterizes many of the songs, the female lead singer of a group named Crowded Head (Brown, 2001), accompanied by a pounding guitar rhythm, offers a frank description of her situation: "Well, you can call me a bitch. . . I've got the post-menstrual blues." There are few verses to the song as it consists mostly of hard guitar riffs and a repetition of the line "I got the pms blues" rhymed with "nothin' to loose." But there is a peculiar detail that suggests that either the singer has an atypical response to her period or that the writer didn't know what the term "pms" actually stood for. Four times in the course of the song she sings, "I've got the post-menstrual cycle blues." The feelings and behavior being identified are commonly associated with a "pre-menstrual" syndrome, not a "post-menstrual" one. But then song writers, like poets, are often allowed a lot of license so this deviation or ignorance of the topic might pass unnoticed.

As mentioned, about half of the songs listed express a male perspective. And just as the woman's songs reflect their own feelings as well as how it affects their relationships with others, the songs from male voices are also sometimes introspective, but most concentrate on how they cope with women and the impact menstrual conditions have upon their lives and feelings.

One of the most original treatments by a male is titled "Double PMS Blues" by Dave Blackledge. The song gives a new spin to the idea of menstrual synchronicity:

My girl friends feelin' bloated
My wife has the cramps
Well it looks like little Willie will be stayin' in my pants. (Blackledge, 2006)

Presumably, the two women with whom he has sexual relationships do not know each other, yet somehow their cycles are in sync with each other so that he has to deal with two sets of mood swings and a double dose of sexual frustration. He goes on to describe them with a clever pun on "cycle" in a way that expresses the notion that women are dangerous and to be avoided during "that time of the month." He compares the two women to "biker chicks" around whom "you can't take any chances."

Unintentionally, the song raises provocative questions about the workings of menstrual synchronicity—the widely held but scientifically unproven idea that women living in close quarters such as dormitories, prisons, and barracks tend to eventually develop fairly synchronous menstrual cycles. Is it conceivable that the two women in this song have somehow linked up their cycles through shared sexual contact with the same man? It will take more than a song writer to answer that question.

The blues singer David Wells offers a similar put-upon view in a song that has the feeling of a dirge and eventually becomes somewhat whiney as he suggests that the woman is "possessed." The song does have a sense of humor (rhyming "possessed" with "egress" is pretty amusing), and toward the end of the piece he suggests a couple of alternative meanings for the letters "pms" that are playful but basically reinforce the "woe is me" view of the man as the innocent target of hormonally induced irrational rage. He asks if "pms" stands for "puffy, moody and sad" or "punish my spouse."

A male lead vocalist in a band named 20 Point Turn (Anon., 2012) offers a full-throated indictment (instructing the guitar to "make it funky now") of how women victimize men by opening with a lyric about how he has to check into a Holiday Inn on a monthly basis. There follows a series of short verses that identify a list of complaints, each one followed by a repetition of the opening reprieve. All of this is accompanied, appropriately, by a reliance on the guitar's wah-wah pedal to capture the petulant tenor of the song. One might even suggest a note of unintended irony in the presence of a would-be macho male striking such a bitchy posture.

Self-indulgence takes another turn at the microphone in Dave Getchell's folksy acoustic guitar performance. Like Dave Blankledge noted previously, Getchell complains about being deprived of sexual pleasure with the implication that it is the woman's rejection of sex during her period rather than his own avoidance that is in play. And Getchell doesn't mention pms but instead alludes to it with the coy phrase "time of the month." It's a study in self pity including the fact that he is not getting any "sweet ectasy tonight."

In contrast, Larry Garner's guitar blues takes the tack of the "sensitive male." Garner recorded his "P.M.S. Blues" song on two different albums, giving each one a different treatment, one with a funky upbeat tempo and the other in a slower Louisiana blues treatment. (Garner, 1998). His character doesn't even want to use the common terms for periodic menstrual mood swings. Rather, he expressed his sympathy with the line, "I get so sad when my baby gets them once-a-month blues." Men in this category are expressing their own version of menstrual synchronicity. They identify so closely with their mate's emotions that they echo the mood swings. It's a male form of menstrual bonding via empathetic mirroring. There's an avuncular quality to the delivery that is framed as giving mature advice to other men who are struggling to understand how to deal with the women in their lives. Toward the end he offers a take on the situation with a positive spin: it could have been worse; she might have missed it. Garner offers a useful perspective: no matter what kinds of moods and problems come with PMS, the arrival of the period is always good news if one wants to avoid pregnancy.

A singer identified as Harmonica Mike offers yet another way of looking at menstrual synchronicity. He opens with a description of hanging out in a bar with a friend describing how bad his girlfriend is behaving and then admits that he too is miserable with his own version of PMS blues (Anon., 2005).

It turns out that many of the songs, both by women and man, take the form of advice or coping suggestions ranging from resignation to avoidance. One of the simplest is found in a song by Dave Thrift who advises that men just have to accept the inevitable and learn to live with it.

And then there are a few instrumental songs on the list that bear the title "P.M.S. Blues" though the performances don't necessarily meet the musical definitions of "blues." For instance, Peter Morgan (Anon., 2012) offers a piece that is dominated by a wailing saxophone, guitar and a stuttering harmonica. One would have to ask the artist what made him associate these sounds with the condition the title alludes to.

The dominant theme throughout these songs, almost without exception, whether expressed by a man or a woman, is some sort of self-pity. Women feel bad about how bad they feel and sometimes feel bad about had bad they make others feel. Men feel bad about how bad the women make them feel or how badly the women treat them. Some men feel bad on behalf of the women but more often just want to stay out of their way. For both men and women menstruation is an alienating phenomenon. Menstrual transactions during this phase of the cycle are fraught with peril and the idea of engaging in sexual activity is unthinkable.

In effect, the views and perspectives expressed throughout popular songs that address menstruation serve to reinforce, with very few exceptions, the most negative stereotypes that are deeply embedded within the culture. This even includes the idea of menstrual isolation, the menstrual hut. But most often it is the men who need to be sent away, preferably to a hotel or bar, to hang out with other men suffering similar banishment while the woman remain at home wallowing in their condition and consuming the prescribed treatments: chocolates and Midol.

Beyond the narrowly prescribed list of songs on the iTunes "P.M.S. Blues" list, there are a few others that are similarly dedicated entirely to exploring some phase of the menstrual cycle. Though it does not show up on the iTunes list being discussed, Mary J. Blige's song titled "PMS" on her early album, *No More Drama*, presents a contrast to Dolly Parton's defiant assessment of the matter. Blige begins her selection by directly inviting the women listening to the song to commiserate then proceeds into a slow, mournful recitation of how miserable she is with the presumption that every woman who hears her has similar feelings. She describes feeling ugly and uncaring about anyone else's problems (Blige, Geter-Tillman, Green, Robinson, & Thompson, 2001).

In the background a chorus of women chant the phrase "pms, pms, pms" in a funereal drone that gives the piece the feeling of abject misery. There is a curious assumption, reinforced by the backup voices and the lyrical claim, that "the worst part of being a woman is PMS," that all women will be able to "relate to" the experience being described. There's something insistent—even a requirement—that all woman have the identical experience, otherwise they lack sufficient sympathy and membership in the menstrual sisterhood.

A similar sense of bonding, though lacking the didactic tone of Blige's song, is expressed by Ani DiFranco in "Blood in The Boardroom" (DiFranco, 1994). The song sketches a dramatic moment when the character in the lyrics is the only woman attending a meeting with a group of men in a corporate office headquarters. She's "sitting in the board room, the I'm so bored room" feeling alienated from the gathering of "suits," a feeling that is magnified by the fact that in the middle of the meeting she gets her period and has to leave to find a toilet. Upon rising she sees that she has left a bloody stain on the white upholstered chair. The experience leads her to philosophize on the meaning of menstruation and to bond with a secretary in the outer office who, of course, offers her a tampon and sympathy.

One of the things that makes this song stand out from all those mentioned so far is that it is a song of praise for menstruation. It sets aside the negative associations while reducing gender differences to essentials. She describes men as having "the instruments of death" as opposed to her ability to "make breath." The song takes some liberties with the biological facts of life in claiming that women "bleed to renew life," given the fact that the onset of menstrual bleeding is an indication that a woman is not pregnant, but as menstrual flow is a reminder of the potential to ovulate and "renew life" the line works on a larger scale by noting the potential to "make life," to "make breath." Apparently the woman in this song has a less onerous relationship with her menstrual life than those cited in the preceding discussion in that she wasn't even aware that her period was imminent. The fact that there is a range of expressions within the oeuvre of menstrual-themed music is a reflection of the range of reactions that the larger population of women in general experience.

At an extreme distance from the positive attitude that Ani DiFranco brings to her period lie two songs that are nasty as well as ignorant of the menstrual facts of life. Eminem's 2002 album *The Eminem Show* includes two brief menstrual details that are sadly revealing. The album consists mainly of a boastful rap about how deprived the Hip-Hop scene must have felt during a time when some personal and legal problems kept Eminem from writing and performing new material. Among the long list of amazing talents and attributes he assigns to himself in a track titled "Without Me," he includes an interesting metaphor, "I'm on the rag and ovulating" (Bass et al., 2002). Now, for a rapper with a notorious record of misogyny to choose ovulation as a means of laying claim to creative and artistic capacity is quite surprising. But to couple ovulation with being "on the rag" is to reveal a fundamental misunderstanding of the workings of the menstrual cycle. Perhaps his desire to find a rhyme for "operating" and "complicating," the words that precede and follow "ovulating" motivated the choice.

Elsewhere on the same album a song titled "Superman" (Bass, King, & Mathers, 2002) consists of little more than a series of violent images and threats aimed at women who have had the audacity to stand up to Slim Shady or expect anything of him. The most ugly image is when he rhymes "anthrax" with "Tampax" and describes using the tampon as a club to beat a woman.

The thought of a deadly poison applied to a feminine hygiene product that will be used as a cudgel is chilling—weaponizing the tampon against its user! Though "anthrax" and "Tampax" do rhyme, associating the two of them is beyond the normal notion of poetic license. There is a sad irony embedded in these details as elsewhere on the album Eminem includes tender, loving references to his young daughter with whom he appears to have a caring relationship.

A more tender approach to the topic of menstruation sung by a male, though the fact that the song is about menstruation is almost completely obscured, is found in a 1954 gospel song written by Sam Cooke and recorded before he became a pop star and was in a group known as The Soul Stirrers. "Touch the Hem of His Garment" (Cooke, 1964) is the retelling of a Biblical story about Jesus and his healing powers, previously discussed in Chapter 2.

Returning to the iTunes listings, it is revealing to observe what shows up on the listings when one broadens the search beyond the "P.M.S. Blues" entries to the word "menstruation." The results are peculiar. Of the 90 items on the list, most are instrumentals and at first it is hard to discern what idea about menstruation motivated the connection. But on closer examination it seems that the common threads are a driving beat with plenty of distorted voices and instruments, a repetitive techno beat or a grunge band sound, all of which leave the impression that there is something frantic and distorting—even deranged—that menstruation brings to mind. Furthermore, the titles of songs and performers under the rubric suggest horror movie associations rather than reproductive glories.

Some representative titles and artists:

"Boiling Menstruation" by Splattered Entrails

"Gargle Upon the Menstruation" by Hemorrhaging Elysium

"Menstruation Sucker" by Absolute disgrace

"Fake Menstruation" by Pooping Poop Poopers

"Menstruation Is the Best Lubrication" by TxPxFx

"Menstruation Glamour" by Felix Kubin

"Sucking the Menstruation" by Splattered Entrails

"Fatal Menstruation" by Death Instincts

"Menstruation and Masturbation" by Pelvs

"Chronic Menstruation" by Lars Carlsson

"F****g Menstruation" by Dani Retamosa & Lorenzo Miguez (The asterisks appear in the list; this item appears 11 times with different album titles; all are in a techno/disco style with no lyrics.)

"Chaotic Cornfuck" by Demented Retarded (This group from the Czech Republic has 17 listings and, due to the distorted Death Metal or Grindcore style it is hard to discern if any of the lyrics include a menstrual element.)

"Menstruation Rite" by Beth Kleist (Though it might seem that this title would make a reference to the cycle, its 1'11 time consists solely of an instrumental drone.)

"Drenched Menstruation" by Limbsplitter

"F**k my Vagina" by Casualties Uv Menstruation

"Purulent Menstruation" by Bigot (An entire two minutes of distortion.)

"Wrecked Menstruation" by Ovulation Mob (Fifty-three seconds of workout beats.)

"Menstruation Cocktail" by Rectal Smegma (1'21(A collection of discordant sounds on an album titled *Keep On Smiling.)*

"Infernal Menstruation" by Otto Von Schirach (Electronic sound effects and beats.)

"Mouthful of Menstruation" by Gorgasm

"Beautiful Parasites" by Menstruation Monsters & Kristall (Three items on the list by this group.)

"The Horse Is Off to Gallup" by Menstruation Sisters

"Menstruation" (There are six entries by separate artists for this title; in neither style nor content do they have any similarity.)

The transgressive style of so many of these songs brings to mind those menstrual activists who flaunt their defiance of the menstrual rules of order by performing what has come to be known as "free bleeding," purposely not using any kind of menstrual management device (tampon, pad, cup, etc.) so that their menstrual blood is allowed to run down their legs, stain their clothing and otherwise become plainly visible. Such "actions" have occurred in a variety of venues, most notably when the marathon runner Kiran Ghandi's participated in the 2015 London marathon claiming that, "she did it to raise awareness about women around the world who have no access to feminine products and to encourage women to not be ashamed of their periods." (Adams, 2015)

Other, more controlled displays have included painting red stains on the back of light colored pants and skirts in order to make the same statement. By assigning menstrual titles to one's musical compositions or to one's band, a similar violation of menstrual norms is accomplished.

There is one more category within the iTunes listings that deserves comment. But, first some background: The 1960 approval by the Food and Drug Administration (FDA) of the oral contraceptive that came to be known as "The Pill" ranks as one of the most life-changing and socially significant scientific developments of the century. Though less dramatic than the discovery of penicillin or the development of nuclear energy and the atomic bomb, its effects on interpersonal relations, sexual behavior, demographic phenomena and a host of other human arrangements has been undeniably profound. And all of the outcomes are the result of the ability to chemically alter the functioning of the menstrual cycle. Furthermore, use of The Pill, though requiring a prescription from a licensed medical doctor, became a highly personal matter. Decisions regarding its use were left to a large degree in the hands of women who, for the first time in history, could gain control of their reproductive cycles.

Much has been written about the impact of The Pill which brings us to ask, in the context of this chapter's concerns, how has it been treated within song lyrics? A search of the iTunes troves under the prompt "the pill" yields 100 items. It is hard to discern what most of them actually have to do with any specific pill. Some refer to album titles that use the word "pill" in a metaphoric way, and many are about drug use such as LSD or other "recreational" substances. Surprisingly, only three of the titles are devoted to the contraceptive pill, but those are revealing.

The most significant is a 1975 release by the country music star, Loretta Lynn. It describes a woman's relationship with her husband who treats her as his brood hen seeing to it that she becomes pregnant every year. But then she discovers the liberating benefits of the pill and it changes her life. It liberates her from her husband's power and opens the world to her (Allen, Bayless, Lynn, & McHan, 1975).

The song develops the hen house metaphor by referring to herself as "this chicken" and mention of the husband's "crowing" and "roostin' time." But it pulls up short of being completely negative toward the man by suggesting that the fact that she's now "got the pill" means, "Oh daddy don't you worry none cause momma's got the pill."

The record became one of Loretta Lynn's most popular singles but also stirred up some controversy, particularly in rural areas dominated by more conservative religious and social values. Due to its enthusiastic endorsement of contraception and celebration of women's sexuality, as well as its bleak view of her husband, some radio stations in the country-western category refused to air it resulting in it getting a lower rank on the play charts than it otherwise might have. Its impact was noteworthy as some doctors in rural areas claimed that the song helped to promote birth control among their women patients (Johnson-Champ, 2012).

The benefits of birth control identified in the lyrics were not limited to relief from child-bearing responsibilities. The ability to manage one's menstrual cycle had additional fashion and life style pay offs (not to mention some creative rhyming opportunities). She describes her new wardrobe by discarding her maternity dress "in the garbage" so she can wear dresses that "won't take up so much yardage."

A male take on the impact of the pill was expressed in a folk song written by a Scottish musician named Matt McGinn and performed by Pete Seeger in his best attempt to replicate a Scottish brogue (McGinn, 1968). The plot line of the song concerns a devout Catholic man's conflict between his sexual desires and his religious commitment to uphold the church's ban on contraception. When he hears stories about the possibility that the Vatican will lift the ban on the pill, he sees it as a belated reprieve. He sings of getting married at the age of 17 with the expectation of having children but that having so many of them became a strain. He went to his priest for advice about controlling his sexual lust (because "my willie was behavin' like a beast") but was scolded because he'd been married for seven years and had only six children. He goes on to reflect on his present situation. Now that he is 40 and has 22 children he is desperately awaiting the Pope's approval of the pill as his wife will be home soon and he knows "his willie" will be undeterred by the fact that his impulse will likely lead to child number 23.

On the surface this song is a lighthearted romp as well as a mild poke at the kind of rigid orthodoxy that can lead to extreme consequences. From the man's point of view it explores the same effects as Loretta Lynn's praise of the pill. In her case she is celebrating the liberation that the pill has brought her while in his it expresses anticipation of another kind of liberation, the ability to engage in sexual activity without the consequences of more burdensome parenthood.

A far darker and politically charged view of the pill and its impact is found in a 1977 composition by a group known as The Last Poets. Founded in 1968 in Harlem on Malcolm X's birthday and credited with having been a shaping influence on the emergence of Hip-Hop, The Last Poets took on a wide range of political issues affecting African-American people as well as geopolitical topics involving race relations across the globe.

At first glance one might not think that the menstrual cycle warranted the attention of civil rights activists or those concerned with racial justice. However, recent drives to eliminate sales tax levies on menstrual products, legislative initiatives to require regulations on product manufacture and content, and efforts to provide free sanitary products to women in prisons, schools, and homeless shelters have demonstrated that menstruation management does indeed have political and economic ramifications, including class and race elements. The perspective that The Last Poets brought to the subject was embedded in a critique of American governmental and philanthropic efforts to initiate modern contraceptive practices into what have come to be called "developing nations," which, in the context of the song's lyrics, are invariably African or Asian, which is to say, non-white. Rather than viewing such efforts as liberating or uplifting, contraceptive devices were viewed as merely another technology of domination. The view is articulated in the opening lines of their song which claim that "its basic design is to kill" (El Hadi, 1977).

In effect, the lyrics equate ovulation control with abortion or even infanticide. The premise is that those advocating the provision of contraception in the form of the pill have an underlying motive: to curtail the increase in demographic groups viewed as undesirable by the ruling (white) culture. And lest there be any doubt as to who the villains are, they are clearly—and crassly—identified as "the hag / With the little black bag."

It is worthy of note that all of the individuals who have been identified with The Last Poets have been men. They have presumed to speak on behalf of members of their racial and class identity as well as for women of color, including those in the regions where contraceptive services were being offered. While the merits of their analysis of the motives behind philanthropic and governmental interventions in other regions deserves consideration, the absence of attention to the desires of those affected by the programs might be seen as arrogant or patronizing. Underlying all of these observations about the social and personal significance of pharmaceutical interventions in the functioning of the menstrual cycle is the unexamined fact that the complete focus is on the workings of women's biology. There has not been a similar effort to find ways to chemically alter sperm production and there are no songs dedicated to the liberating effects of vasectomies. Once again, as in other facets of the definitions, management, and social construction of menstruation, the transactional nature of the experience results in men playing a dominant role in the outcomes. Just as men were the inventors of the pill and the members of the regulatory agencies that determined its approval and conditions of prescription, they have also been instrumental in shaping its social perception and employment.

Or, to express the matter in a musical metaphor, though menstruation is a solo performance and every woman produces her own unique rhythm according to the composition of her body's orchestration, the performance is in accordance with the traditions of its oeuvre. And though men lack the instrument necessary to play the tune, they share in creating the conditions of its reception. The collaboration is sometimes harmonious and sometimes discordant. It's an awkward duet.

Note

All of the songs discussed were located on the iTunes web site and the lyrics were transcribed from downloads of the songs. The following set of citations refers to recorded versions of the songs that are available, according to the publishers. However, there are likely to be discrepancies between versions available on recordings and those on the web site. Furthermore, it was not possible to locate recorded versions for several of the songs which could only be found on the iTunes site.

References

Adams, C. (August 13, 2015). Runner defends letting period bleed freely at London Marathon. *People*. Retrieved on November 5, 2018 from http://people.com/celebrity/kiran-gandhi-period-runner-speaks-out-against-critics/

Allen, L., Bayless, T. D., Lynn, L., & McHan, D. (1975). The Pill [Recorded by Loretta Lynn]. On *Back to the Country* [Record]. Mt. Juliet, TN: Bradley's Barn.

Anon. (2003). PMS [Recorded by American Gypsy]. On *Let Me Be...Free* [CD]. Team 3 productions.

Anon. (2007). PMS [Recorded by Cherri & The Violators]. On *First Offense* [CD]. Dilligas Publishing.

Anon. (2005). PMS Blues [Recorded by Harmonica Mike & The Delta Heat]. On *Blues...From Baton Rogue* [CD]. Baton Rouge, LA: East Studios.

Anon. (2012). PMS Blues [Recorded by 20 Point Turn]. On *Dirt Floor Party* [CD]. Reverb-nation.

Bass, J., Bell, K., Dudley, A., Horn, T., Mathers, M., & McLaren, M. (2002). Without Me. [Recorded by Eminem]. On *Without Me* [CD]. 54 Studios, Encore Studios.

Bass, J., King, S., & Mathers, M. (2002). Superman. [Recorded by Eminem, feat. Dina Rae]. On *The Eminem Show* [CD]. Santa Monica, CA: Interscope/Aftermath Records.

Blackledge, D. (2006). Double PMS Blues. [Recorded by Dave Blackledge]. On *Spread It on Thick* [CD]. David J. Blackledge.

Blige, M., Geter-Tillman, T., Green, A., Robinson, T., & Thompson, C. (2001). PMS. [Recorded by Mary J. Blige]. On *No More Drama* [CD]. MCA Records.

Brown, P. (2001). PMS Blues [Recorded by Crowded Head]. On *Voices* [CD]. New York, NY: Orchard Records.

Budway, K. (2000). PMS Blues [Recorded by Kathy & Shanti]. On *Time to Move On*. Kathy and Shanti Records.

Cooke, S. (1964). Touch the Hem of His Garment [Recorded by Sam Cooke]. On *Sam Cooke with the Soul Stirrers* [Record]. Fantasy.

Cooper, A., & Wagner, D. (1975). Only Women Bleed [Recorded by Alice Cooper]. On *Only Women Bleed* [CD]. Atlantic Records.

Daniels, L., Emile, D., Jerkins, R., & Yasin, T. (2007). Feedback [Recorded by Janet Jackson]. On *Discipline* [MP3]. Atlantic City, NJ: 2nd Floor Studios.

DiFranco, A. (1993). Blood in The Boardroom [Recorded by Ani DiFranco]. On *Puddle Dive* [CD]. Buffalo, NY: Righteous Babe Records.

El Hadi, S. (1977). The Pill [Recorded by The Last Poets]. On *Delights of the Garden* [Record]. Charly Records.

Garner, L. (1998). PMS [Recorded by Larry Garner]. On *Standing Room Only* [CD]. Memphis, TN: Ardent Studios.

Getchell, D. (2004). PMS Blues [Recorded by Dave Getchell]. On *A Slant on Life and Living* [CD]. Frontiers of Freedom.

Johnson-Champ, D. (2012). On the 40th anniversary of Loretta Lynn's "The Pill," women are still fighting the battle for contraception. Retrieved on November 5, 2012 from http://addictinginfo.com/2012/02/20/on-the-40th-anniversary-of-loretta-lynns-the-pill-women-are-still-fighting-the-battle-for-contraception-video/

McGinn, M. (1968). The Pill [Recorded by Pete Seeger]. On *A Link in the Chain* [CD]. Legacy/Sony Music Distribution.

Morgan, P. (2012). PMS 286 Blues [Recorded by Peter Morgan]. On *Looky Hear* [MP3]. Pacific Audio Records.

Noll, C. (2014). PMS Blues. Retrieved on November 5, 2018 from https://www.youtube.com/watch?v=JqpqT-kvCts

Parton, D. (1994). PMS Blues [Recorded by Dolly Parton]. On *Heartsongs: Live from Home* [CD]. Celebrity Theatre, Dollywood: Columbia Records.

Thrift, D. (2006). PMS Blues [Recorded by Dave Thrift]. On *Blues Extreme* [CD]. Dave Thrift Records.

Wells, D. (2007). PMS [Recorded by Dave Wells]. On *Deeper Shade of Blue* [CD]. Amazon Music.

CHAPTER NINE

Menstrual Mischief and Transgressions

Woe to the hand that shed this costly blood!...
Let but the commons hear this testament,
Which, pardon me, I do not mean to read,
And they would kiss dead Caesar's wounds,
And dip their napkins in his sacred blood,
Yea, beg a hair of him for memory,
And dying, mention it within their wills,
Bequeathing it as a rich legacy
Unto their issue.

> Marc Anthony
> Shakespeare, *Julius Caesar*, Act III, Scene 2

Mark Anthony's lines capture one view of a particular kind of blood loss: arterial blood that has been shed in the service of one's country; blood lost in martyrdom; blood that is so valuable as to be worthy of being soaked up and preserved as a cherished memento. This view echoes the veneration given Christ's blood as expressed in numerous stories, songs, and images. In fact, the belief in the concept of transubstantiation is so strong that once communion wine has been blessed and transformed into blood, priests have been known to fall upon the floor to lick up any of the fluid that has accidentally spilled from the chalice. The belief in the power of the blood of Christ is so strong that the greatest wish of many Christians is to be "washed in the blood" of Christ.

Similarly, in an echo of the practice that Anthony prescribed, members of the Calabrian Mafia in Italy are so dedicated to the leaders of the clan that, "More than once, they had been seen rushing to the corpse of an assassinated boss, dipping a handkerchief in his blood, and pressing it to their lips" (Perry, 2018, p. 40).

Menstrual blood, in contrast, is also often seen as powerful but at the other end of the value spectrum. While arterial blood is venerated, menstrual blood is commonly treated with fear and disgust, shunned and discarded in secrecy. In some cultures, contact with it, especially by men, is a deeply ingrained taboo. Men will even deprive themselves of sexual pleasure rather than come in contact with the substance.

However, just as arterial blood has been assigned a rich variety of symbolic meanings and applications too numerous to list here, menstrual blood has also received symbolic and metaphoric treatments, although much more subtle.

Anthropologists, psychologists, philosophers and others have explored the cultural significance of menstruation and the reasons for menstrual taboos. Some have studied the bases of the taboos (e.g., Durkheim, 1915), the origins of attitudes (e.g., Douglas, 1966), the variety of management practices across cultures (e.g., Mead, 1928; Buckley & Gottlieb, 1988; Mead, 1928), psychic significance (e.g., Bettelheim, 1962), economic role (e.g., Knight, 1991), symbolic uses in literature (e.g., Medoro, 2002), and any number of other aspects of the complex responses (mostly negative) to the presence of menses in cultural contexts.

From ancient writers such as Aristotle, Galen, and Pliney to popular culture products such as the Comedy Central series, *South Park* (see Chapter 5 for full discussion), there has been an endless stream of efforts to assail the daunting task of attributing meaning to the menstrual phenomenon. They have yielded a vast array of "cultural response[s] to the physically extraordinary," to borrow an apt expression from Buckley and Gottlieb (1988, p. 46); one of the most extreme is captured in the joke that expresses male estrangement, "Never trust anything that can bleed for seven days and not die."

But wherever there are taboos, there are breakers of taboos, or, as a colloquial expression would have it, "Laws are made to be broken." While much has been written about the nature of the menstrual rules of order and what the consequences of breaking the laws might be (cleansing rituals, temporary banishment, etc.), there has been no systematic study of how women have defied the taboos, what motivated them to do so, how men responded and what the consequences were. It turns out that the ways and means of menstrual transgression have been remarkably creative and varied. To some extent this should not be surprising given the complexity of the rules themselves, but it is also a tribute to the power of the taboos that tales of their defiance are more rare than tales of their compliance.

Animal behaviorists have identified a variety of ways that different species lay claim to territory, announce their presence or use their bodies (and the products of their bodies) to communicate with others. Barking, growling, snarling, spitting, whinnying, snorting, thumping, cooing, whistling, purring, roaring, neighing, peeping, cheeping, hissing, baying, scratching, pawing, bristling, crouching, puffing up, rolling over, lying down, turning tail, baring fangs, squinting, and rearing are some of the communications techniques used by animals, and most have some equivalent form in humans. Urine also serves an important signaling function as discussed in Jana Murphy's *The Secret Lives of Dogs* (2000) where she points out that dogs manage a delicate three-legged balancing act in order to aim their stream as high as possible on the fire hydrant or tree in order to impress other sniffers with how big they are. Young boys commonly compete in a similar way and a visitor to high school boys' bathrooms will often notice a row of unflushed urinals where boys have left behind the yellow puddles testifying to their having been there. In *Never Cry Wolf* (1963) the Canadian naturalist Farley Mowat amusingly recounts his own territorial marking experience during his long sojourn in the northern territories while researching the lives of wolves. He drank quarts of tea and proceeded to hike around the hills pissing on shrubs to see if the wolves would respect his territorial claims (They did).

Aside from isolated and rare references in the occasional story, film or personal anecdote, little has been written about the use of menstrual blood or paraphernalia for communicative purposes. Yet there is nothing so well suited for the expression of defiance, transgression, or assertion of one's presence as either literal or symbolic displays of the period.

The following discussion identifies several of the ways that the period has been used as an expressive medium and the purposes in doing so. And virtually all constitute the kind of transaction that either defines or challenges gender relationships.

As discussed previously, when the character in the memoir and film *To Sir, With Love* was faced with an act of menstrual mischief, a used pad smoldering in a classroom heater, it so nearly traumatized him that he invoked a set of naming rituals in order to reassert the gender norms that were essential to his identity as well as his role as a male teacher. His certainty that a girl was responsible for the prank and what shook him to the core was that the menstrual order of things, or what Sophie Laur (1990) calls "menstrual etiquette," has been disturbed, and therefore, by implication, the moral and gender order of the world.

Just as the Biblical patriarch Laban had to reassert the masculine role in the face of his daughter Rachel's menstrual transgression (discussed in Chapter 2), so do contemporary men insist on proper menstrual decorum, as demonstrated in an episode of an MTV reality show called *Sorority Life* (Myers, 2003). The episode involved a sorority and its matched fraternity playing a series of pledge week pranks on each other, escalating to a culminating incident. The boys had just trashed the girls' sorority house with bags of lawn debris and the girls decided to retaliate. One of the girls narrating the story says, "We had to think of something to top them. Like, what's the grossest thing you can think of that would make a guy like so grossed out more than anything? Obviously, tampons! Guys hate them."

The scene proceeds to show the girls unwrapping a number of tampons, soaking them in water then dousing them with ketchup and tuna fish oil. In the middle of the night they drive to the fraternity house, leap out of the car, twirl the tampons in the air and throw them on the porch and bushes in front of the house before leaping back in the car and speeding away. A boy comes out on the porch and calls to his frat mates that the girls have attacked, but when he sees the bloody looking tampons he shakes his head and retreats back inside. The scene closes with two on-camera comments, one from a girl and the other from the boy who saw the tampons:

Girl: "I think boys play harder but they aren't really that smart. I mean, we definitely have a lot better ideas than they do."

Boy: "Pranks have, at least in my book, a clear line and you cross that line and it's just disrespectful. It's done; it's over; no more." (Myers, 2003)

When I first saw this clip, I was startled by the moment when a girl pours tuna fish oil over the tampons. It struck me as an appalling and sad expression of self-loathing. However, I have since discussed the scene with a number of women, many in their 20's, and have been surprised to hear an opposite response. Rather than expressing a negative self-image, women have contended that the tuna oil detail is a frontal attack on the nasty image the boys have of women: "So you think we smell bad?!?! Well, then smell this!!" It certainly is assertive. Whether it asserts confidence or constitutes a confirmation of existing attitudes of menstrual disgust is still an open question, but the program ends with the impression that the girls have bested the boys, or as they might say, "Blood Rules!!"

The line running from the Biblical Rachel to the girls in the sorority house is unswerving. Both fully comprehended the power of the taboos that shape gender relations and applied a kind of reverse spin to turn the power of the taboo back against the men who hold the negative values, thereby threatening the men with contamination. The boy who turns away from the seemingly bloody tampon stuck in the shrubs on his lawn, returning to the safety of his frat mates indoors, is reenacting Laban's retreat to the safe company of the men outside Rachel's tent. Both have been defeated by an act of menstrual aggression. The only significant difference over the millennia is the brazenness of the girls in the sorority. They have invented a strategic use of the dreaded period, their own "WMD," Weapons of Menstrual Destruction.

A similar gesture appeared in the women's marches that took place across America and in other countries following Donald Trump's inauguration. As a means of protesting Trump's tendency to mock or belittle women, particularly his disdainful remark about Megan Kelly following one to the pre-election debates, many women carried signs and images that referred directly to women's reproductive organs and to menstruation.

Clearly, menstrual mischief is not limited to literary and media invention, to times gone by or to political activism. Consider another example of covert hostility that I was told about that occurs in girls' schools in Japan. It seems that if a male teacher is strongly disliked by the girls, it sometimes happens that a used sanitary pad will be stuffed into his shoe in the rack inside the schoolhouse door where outdoor shoes are left upon entering the building. The fact that the teacher's foot has been in contact with the contaminating object and that, furthermore, he must handle it to remove it, humiliates the teacher and becomes a medium for conveying the low regard his students (or at least one of them) have for him. As Sigmund Freud (1913), Margaret Mead (1949) and the 15th chapter of Leviticus have made clear, the nature of the menstrual taboo is such that even if the violation of the taboo was unintentional, the result is stigmatizing. Freud describes the stigma this way: "The strangest fact seems to be that anyone who has transgressed one of these prohibitions himself acquires the characteristic of being prohibited—as though the whole of the dangerous charge had been transferred over to him" (p. 22).

Other school incidents I have been told of are more like "acting out" expressions. I think of them as "menstrual graffiti":

At a private girls' school in New York it would sometimes happen that someone would leave a used tampon dangling from the hook on the inside of a cubicle door. It seems unlikely that the girl who secretly flaunted her period is this manner would know the member of the janitorial staff who had to clean up her menstrual vandalism, but the act suggests a need to assert her gender in ways that both defy and embody the negative conditioning she had experienced.

At another school the girls would sometimes soak tampons in water, twirl them by their strings like the Biblical David swinging his sling shot, and fling them at the ceiling where they would stick and hang like an array of dangling

stalactites. Here the girls are creating a semi-public display of their menstrual paraphernalia in such a way that some representative of the adult, school authorities
must deal with.

These examples have several elements in common. The acts are carried out
anonymously; they are aggressive in nature; and, they are done in recognition of
the fact that "the other" (boys, men, authority, adults) will be disgusted or offended
or have to "clean up" the women's "filth," thereby transferring the onus of "the
curse," the taboo, to an "innocent" other.

An even more aggressive act of menstrual hostility—in this case it becomes
menstrual malice—is described in a novel by Joyce Carol Oates, *The Tattooed Girl*
(2003). Alma Busch, the abused and disturbed girl of the title, is doing household
chores for a man who has been kind to her and who she has no reason to hate or
even dislike, except that he belongs to the gender that has mistreated her all her
life. At one point she is helping to prepare a beef stew dinner for her employer and
a guest, and she repeatedly puts her fingers into her vagina, captures her menstrual
blood and mixes it into the food before serving it. Her transgression is unknown
to the men who consume the food. It apparently does them no harm, and at first
the detail seems to illustrate the depth of her self-loathing and of her similarly
deep-seated hatred of men. However, on a subtler level, this covert act of hostility
also represents one of Alma's first attempts to take charge of her own body and to
strike out against the gender of those who have used and abused her. It is a harbinger of a later scene when she finds the courage to fight back against a man whom
she had thought of as her lover but who had pimped her to others and regularly
abused her. Appropriately, her act of rebellion and self-assertion is to kick him
between the legs.

Furthermore, at the level of symbolic literary analysis, Alma is enacting a
bizarre and twisted travesty of the communion ritual, a crude parody in which
the serving of her menstrual blood to the men enacts her own "last supper." It
is shortly after this event that she begins to shake off her passive acceptance of
her victim status and to assert her new identity as comforting aide to her slowly
failing employer. Her malicious use of her own menstrual blood becomes her
first stumbling step toward her own resurrection as an independent, assertive
woman.

Among the most overt and directly confrontational examples of menstrual
aggression is the previously mentioned story of Donita Sparks, a member of the
punk band L-7, who threw her tampon at some unruly men in an audience (see
Chapter 1). The public display of private parts has long been recognized as a male
act of aggression, and Germaine Greer has argued in *The Whole Woman* (1999)
that there is no female counterpart since men like women to expose themselves so

mooning and flashing are in fact signs of submission when performed by women. Greer claims that, "Though male genital exposure frightens women, female genital exposure, whether intended to be hostile or alluring, reinforces men's sense of their own superiority. As long as men think of women's bodies as commodities offered for their consumption, there is no liberation to be had either in taking clothes off or in keeping bodies covered" (p. 198).

But the flaunting of a unique *product* of the female reproductive organs, menstrual blood soaked into a tampon, turns the power formulation on its head. Just as it is believed that women do not welcome the uninvited display of male sexual organs because the act implies an expression of the gendered power differential, the unwelcome display of the period (and it is *always* unwelcome except when it denotes that one has been spared an unwanted pregnancy) denotes a woman's rejection of the customary shame and embarrassment through which she has been conditioned to accept her role. The outrageousness of this act parodies the well-established custom of male performers such as James Brown, Willie Nelson and a long list of others, who commonly throw their sweat soaked handkerchiefs or bandannas to their (female) fans.

While most of the examples noted so far have been expressions of rejection of the menstrual rules of etiquette, sometimes menstrual mischief takes on a creative or even friendly aspect as in this example. It concerns a woman who, upon graduating from college in the mid-1970's moved back to the small town she grew up in, away from the circle of friends and a lover whom she missed badly. One day during her period she took a post card, smeared a streak of menstrual blood across it and mailed it to her distant boy friend. She explains the act as both a symbolic defiance of the U.S. Government as personified by the postal system (the woman was an ardent anti-war activist) and as a way of sharing the intimacy of her period with her lover. The "message" she was sending negated one set of rules while secretly asserting in a positive fashion her erotic playfulness.

So far, I have been focusing only on cases in which individuals have used actual menstrual blood or products as a medium for the expression of some sort of dissent, transgression or defiance. However, the menstrual taboo is so strong that merely mentioning the subject can demonstrate the speaker's willingness to defy authority, mainly the authority of the patriarchal taboo itself. The idea of bringing the period into the open for purposes of either upsetting the status quo or reinforcing it can apply to both men and women. And it frequently finds expression in the realm of humor via passing remarks, jokes, skits, and even extended plot lines in movies and TV shows. This brings us to the subject of menstrual humor.

There are a number of theories regarding humor—what makes us laugh. One particular kind of humor is sometimes described as "at the expense of" or "making fun of" someone else, some "other" who is the "butt" of the joke, who is mocked, shamed or made to look ridiculous, even suffering injury as the in the plethora of You Tube postings of people having accidents of various kinds and at whose misfortune we giggle and take pleasure. One explanation for this sort of laughter is that we're relieved that we're not the ones being exposed, embarrassed or hurt by some cruel twist of fate. We realize that "it could have been me," and laughter expresses our fleeting pleasure at having been spared the existential misfortune that "the other" is enduring.

Menstrual humor entails layers of possibilities and potential pitfalls for both men and women who attempt to express it, be it in a casual social remark, as a stand-up comic or within a dramatic story line. Its use and permissibility have evolved just as have other topics that were at one time open game for laughter but which later became off limits. Race-based humor has gone through such a transformation. It was once common for white comics to include jokes with racist themes and the history of minstrel shows demonstrates how acceptable it was at one time for white performers to build an entire sub-genre of theater around racial stereotypes. Today, the only comics who include race material in their acts are those like Dave Chappelle who has based some of his most effective pieces on how both white and black people construct narrow notions of race and imbue them with social consequences. Chappelle can use the kind of loaded, offensive language that would likely curtail the career of a white comic.

Similarly, menstrual humor has become pretty much the sole province of women comics—with a few exceptions. A skit by the comedy duo Jordan Peele and Keegan-Michael Key on their Comedy Central show *Key & Peele* was titled, "Menstruation Orientation" (2015). It depicted two men giving a "sensitivity lecture" in the form of a TED Talk to an audience full of men about how to behave with the women in their lives when they were menstruating. The script is risky, full of lines about the importance of "being nice to your bitches," but it's also very funny and captures a lot of what makes menstruation feel like such a foreign and frightening thing to many men.

Meanwhile, in keeping with the tendency to build comic material around mention of one's own life drama, including the humiliations and disappointments one encounters (consider Louis C.K.'s bits about his own masturbation practices), women have delved into their personal menstrual histories for material that was often disturbing or emotionally painful but in the retelling while standing behind a microphone before a comedy club or theater audience becomes worthy of laughter. The source of the laughter is often little more than the catharsis of sharing, knowing that many members of the audience, at least the women in the room, have had—or have feared—a similar encounter. And encounters they often are, menstrual transactions, incidents that were deeply embedded in shared but previously not publically acknowledged conditioning and folklore.

In response to male use of menstrual jokes and insults as a put down, women have developed ways to use menstrual references to mock men, to make them squirm in their discomfort at being confronted with the menstrual realities of life and to lay claim to their own histories and perspectives as worthy of attention. Probably the most famous example of such an expression was Gloria Steinem's essay, "If Men Could Menstruate" published in 1978 in *Ms. Magazine*. The essay unpacks the nature of menstrual taboos and secrecy by suggesting that men would boast about their flow and celebrate each cycle.

As long as the social construction of gender continues to be a contested matter (and there is no sign that those definitions will ever be settled) every aspect of human biology that gets layered with signification, be it breasts, penis, sperm, menses, vagina, or the secondary, social characteristics such as hair style, grooming, clothing, shoes, etc., there will be efforts to challenge the assignments through humor, politics, and both overt and covert aggression. And it is important to note that the preceding discussion focused exclusively on Western cultures. I cannot possibly do justice to how menstrual transactions play out in other settings. But one example of menstrual transgression in rural India might serve to illustrate how varied the manifestations can be.

Because of the power thought to inhere in a bloody menstrual rag, women have been known to throw their used rag into the street so that anyone who stepped over it had an evil cast put upon them. "The piece of cloth/rag/pad used for menstrual bleeding is considered by rural Indian women as one of the most vulnerable objects and potent agents which might be used for casting evil eyes/magic on someone" (Singh, 2006, p. 11).

Film, Music and Television References

Clavell, J. (Producer & Director). (1967). *To Sir, with Love* [Motion Picture]. United States: Columbia Pictures.

Key, K., & Peele, J. (Creators). (2015). *Key & Peele*. [Television Series]. United States: Comedy Central.

Myers, S. (Creator). (2003). *Sorority Life*. [Television Series]. United States: MTV.

Parker, T., & Stone, M. (Creators). (1997). *South Park*. [Television Series]. United States: Comedy Central.

Print References

Anon. (March, 2007). You have to see this. *Harper's Magazine*, 22–23.

Bettelheim, B. (1962). *Symbolic wounds: Puberty rites and the envious male.* New York, NY: Collier.

Braithwaite, E. R. (1959). *To sir, with love.* New York, NY: Jove Books.

Buckley, T., & Gottlieb, A. (Eds.). (1988). *Blood magic: The anthropology of menstruation.* Berkeley, CA: University of California Press.

Douglas, M. (1966). *Purity and danger: An analysis of concepts of pollution and taboo.* London: Routledge.

Durkheim, E. (1915). *The elementary forms of the religious life.* (Translated by J. W. Swain). London: George Allen & Unwin.

Freud, S. (1913). *Totem and taboo: Resemblances between the psychic lives of savages and neurotics.* New York, NY: Penguin.

Greer, G. (1999). *The whole woman.* New York, NY: Anchor Books.

Houppert, K. (1999). *The curse: Confronting the last unmentionable taboo: menstruation.* New York, NY: Farrar, Straus & Giroux.

Knight, C. (1991). *Blood relations: Menstruation and the origins of culture.* New Haven, CT: Yale University Press.

Laur, S. (1990). *Issues of blood: the politics of menstruation.* London: Palgrave Macmillan.

Mean, M. (1928). *Coming of age in Samoa.* New York: Morrow Quill.

Mead, M. (1949). *Male and female.* New York, NY: William Morrow.

Medoro, D. (2002). *The bleeding of America: Menstruation as symbolic economy in Pynchon, Faulkner, and Morrison.* Westport, CT: Greenwood Press.

Mowat, F. (1963). *Never cry wolf.* Toronto: McClelland and Stewart.

Murphy, J. (2000). *The secret lives of dogs: The real reasons behind 52 mysterious canine behaviors.* New York, NY: Rodale Books.

Oates, J. (2003). *The tattooed girl.* New York, NY: Harper Collins.

Perry, A. (January 22, 2018). Blood and justice. *The New Yorker, 40,* 36–47.

Singh, A. J. (January-March 2006). The place of menstruation in the reproductive lives of women of rural North India. *Indian Journal of Community Medicine, 31*(1), 10–14.

CHAPTER TEN

Random Menstrual Moments

One of the things that makes the social construction of menstruation a topic of inexhaustible interest is the random ways it makes its presence felt. Every cultural, every era, and every religion has crafted its own unique perspective and body of lore to define and confine this elusive and mysterious biological fact of life. There will never be a comprehensive, all-inclusive encyclopedia (or Wikipedia) of menstruation because its meaning is in a constant state of flux. Therefore, in order to provide a few more glimpses, snapshots, as it were, of the diverse nature of the subject, the following "menstrual sightings" are intended to demonstrate the diversity of menstrual transactions that exist.

The Manopause Defense

Male attempts to appropriate for their own purposes traits associated with women can assume some truly weird dimensions. In July 2006 the Hollywood star Mel Gibson, who was 57 years old at the time, was stopped at a checkpoint in a routine traffic procedure. According to reports of the incident, when officers insisted that he show them his driver's license, which he did not have with him, he flew into a rage and accused the police of harassing him. He was arrested for driving under the influence (DWI) and in the course of the encounter he was recorded making several anti-Semitic remarks. (Gardner, 2013)

On another occasion, following a heated argument with a girlfriend, Gibson wrote a letter to her explaining that his violent temper was a result of his undergoing male menopause. According to reports, the letter stated, "I don't know why I'm so whacky and depressed but I need to get well and re-enter life. Maybe it's some kind of male menopause" (Freeman, 2010).

The Gibson stories gave rise to a flurry of tabloid pieces and social media posts about whether or not men experienced changes induced by age-related hormonal fluctuations, sometimes known as testosterone deficiency, androgen deficiency, and late-onset hypogonadism. For instance, Yvonne Fulbright, an on-air reporter for the Fox news network who is known as the "Foxsexpert" stated, under a headline reading, "NOT SUCH A MYTH: MALE MENO-PAUSE": (2009).

> He's feeling hot flashes—and they have nothing to do with desire. Like a woman, his body is letting him know it's going through "male menopause." Far from being a myth, this hotly debated experience really does exist. Yet few people know about the condition more formally known as andropause.

The existence of this newly noted malady, though it is not listed in the *Diagnostic and Statistical Manual of Mental Disorders* (DSM-5), the document used to define and justify medical coverage for psychiatric conditions, has been gaining traction. In 1998 a book titled *Male Menopause* by Jed Diamond attempted to put men's life changes on a par with women's by claiming that the purpose of the changes men underwent was "to signal the end of First Adulthood and prepare men for Second Adulthood." Apparently the book provoked sufficient interest that a sequel was published a few years later titled, *Surviving Male Menopause: A Guide for Women and Men* (2000). Use of the frightening term "surviving" suggests that there are circumstances in which one might *not* survive the dreaded condition, however, that outcome is not mentioned. Ten years later the author took his argument to yet another level and gave the condition a new name in a book titled, *Mr. Mean: Saving Your Relationship from the Irritable Male Syndrome* (2010). Suggesting a link between hormone-based male behavior with the condition known as "irritable bowel syndrome" may be clever but it hardly elicits sympathy.

There are also numerous web sites dedicated to explaining the condition. The symptoms of the condition commonly include declining sex drive, forgetfulness, weight gain, hair loss, and irritability. In other words, what was once called "getting old" has been given a new identity modeled after a specific set of biological changes that women experience.

As he moves from Road Warrior to Andropause Man, it appears that Mel Gibson has embraced his new role. According to reports in the celebrity press, in addition to the apology cited above, he has also speculated about the reasons he cut back on his screen acting and became a director, "I'll still do the best damn job I can, but it doesn't mean the same thing. I'm going to get the answer for myself one of these days. It's the male menopause, that's what it is" (Anon., 2009).

Aside from its recognizing erectile dysfunction as a treatable condition, the medical establishment has not endorsed andropause as a fully articulated diagnosis with behavioral and/or physiological characteristics comparable to those associated with women's aging. However, it seems inevitable that the present trend will continue and expand. It may be only a matter of time before bad moods in boys and men will be excused as a new version of PMS—Pre-MANstrual Syndrome. Such is the function of menstrual envy.

"The M-Word" (No Longer) on a Movie Screen Near You[1]

It is not clear where the coy linguistic practice of using-while-not-using so called offensive words by appending the term "word" after its initial letter and preceded by "the" came from ("the n-word," "the c-word," "the f-word," "the r-word"). The practice functions in speech the way the "bleep" does on television. Everyone is assumed to know what the word is and says it to oneself, but a quaint regard for a Victorian notion of what can be said in "polite company" allows the word to be put into play while not offending anyone. Furthermore, the construction is usually reserved for talking *about* the word rather than using it in its actual grammatical form. As such, it functions as a meta-phrasing, raising consciousness about the need to be sensitive regarding the potential that words have to hurt or defame their referents.

The director Henry Jaglom has cleverly appropriated the practice by applying it to another value-laden, emotionally charged topic: menopause. And while the word "menopause" itself is not as socially verboten as are the four words alluded to above, menopause itself may be more culturally vexed and discomforting than are race, gender, sex, and cognitive disability which the other coded expressions allude to.

Jaglom's decision to name the film (his 19th feature) *The M-Word* (Marks & Jaglom, 2014) cleverly appropriates the semantic maneuver to several ends. He invites us to think about the function of the hyphenation gambit in all its manifestations while at the same time bringing menstruation out of its closet for some close scrutiny. The plot device employed for this purpose is a "film-within-a-film" construction somewhat similar to that employed in *The Truman Show, The Artist,* and particularly in *Boogie Nights* where the nature of the medium itself and the way

it shapes the behavior of individuals as well as reflecting some of the social circumstances that the film comments on becomes both metaphor and content. In this
case a woman sets out to make a documentary film that involves interviewing a
variety of women (and one man) about their experiences and views on menopause
for a film to be titled, "The M-Word," which is the same as the title of the fictional
film that we're watching.

The film also includes a good deal of commentary on PMS as the women
being interviewed comment on that experience as well and the documentarian in
the film experiences extremely painful menstrual cramps. The main character,
Moxie, is an actor on a children's television show at the fictional KZAM network
in Los Angeles, where the staff seem to have one thing in common: most of them
are menopausal women. The appropriately named Moxie pitches her idea for
"The M Word" at a crucial time—her station is bleeding money and a New York–
based "suit," Charlie Moon (Michael Imperioli), is flown in to assess the situation
(someone is embezzling funds from the station) and make necessary employee
cuts. And this is where the title's second meaning comes into play: money. The
parallel between the menopausal women and the "menopausal" television station
is obvious: both are on their last legs and losing to younger and fresher women/
programming. The discussions about money are handled in the same delicate way
as menopause; it is something no one wants to talk about but everyone knows what
is happening. Moxie, however, brings both M-words out of the closet.

The documentary includes many zany exchanges, as when Moxie asks her
mother "What are you feeling right now?" and her mother (Frances Fisher),
experiencing a hot flash, fans herself with a head of romaine lettuce and responds,
"I'm feeling quite wet." But it is this type of pep that serves Moxie well when
she organizes an impromptu sit-in to save her colleagues' jobs immediately after
Charlie fires a good portion of the staff. By this time a romance has developed
between Moxie and Charlie that pits menopause against money with—spoiler
alert—both coming out victorious in the end. The film also includes a good deal
of commentary on PMS, as the menopausal women interviewed in the documentary reflect on their experiences as younger women. (These interview shots
are humorously intercut with a scene of a debilitated Moxie struggling with her
cramps.) Making the comparison between the painful menstrual cramps they
used to have and the effects of menopause they are currently experiencing, the
film presents the women as now free to enjoy their lives as older women and to
face menopause as a rebirth.

A third M-word that Jaglom toys with refers to the current state of broadcast "Media" with its penchant for sensational and cheap—both in taste and
cost—television content. Charlie is interested in the "reality TV" style of Moxie's

menopause documentary, which is shot on location with hand held cameras and uses non-professional actors. Charlie also identifies its suitability for niche market cable TV, seeing it as a more crass version of programming on the Oprah Channel. The result is a triple M-word send up: menopause, money, media. Unfortunately, the burden of carrying all this baggage is a bit much for what is at bottom a romantic comedy. The improvisational freedom Jaglom allows his actors gives them free rein to banter and top each other's performances, and the film's ambition stretches the run-time to an exhausting two hours that crosses into self-indulgence. Yet despite its limitations, the fact that *The M Word* challenges menstrual taboos and sheds a bit of light on their social construction deserves a nod of respect.

Boxing and Bleeding[2]

In the boxing ring, droplets of blood are often an indication of triumph. In fact, if you've ever had the opportunity to fight, seeing blood on an opponent's face will often evoke a primal, animalistic pleasure. Boxing is, arguably, one of very few scenarios where bleeding is encouraged. In this sport, the notion of blood is a funny thing, depending on where it's coming from. When I sit in my corner after Round 2 of a fight and stare across the ring at my opponent's bloodied face, my trainer encourages me with zeal. Even my own blood, running down my nose and into my mouth is somewhat appealing, reminding me of the warrior I am trained to be. At my boxing club, the carpet lining the ring is stained with visible traces of bloody bouts and sparring. We can point and laugh at whose blood is whose and remember the victory and triumph that resulted from those stains. However, that blood-induced pride would quickly dissipate had it resulted from menstruation.

In the gym, menstruation is held to a sort of "don't ask, don't tell" policy, considering the culture is a male-dominated one. As such, my monthly menstruation is never discussed, unless it's being referred to as disruptive or disgusting. In the boxing community, we encounter a clear and evident divide between that of "good" and "bad" blood: Arterial blood gushing from the nose and face—GOOD! Menstrual blood—BAD! and, further, DISMISSED! Blood will spew and spatter from trauma to the head and fall gracefully onto the ring carpet. It will glaze down an opponent's face and merely be wiped off by the fighter's trainer without any disruption or inconvenience. In contrast, On the heaviest days of menstrual flow, women are in a constant state of alert regarding leakage, running to the bathroom to change a tampon, and of course clean up the mess all alone in shame.

As a female boxer, I thought about my blood on a fairly regular basis. Bleeding is something that should innately occur to my system every 28 days (more or less). However, excessive physical exertion, brief periods of starvation, and rapid weight loss had induced amenorrhea. This is all fancy jargon that basically communicates one simple fact: I don't get a period—ever. For four years, I did not menstruate, and subsequently experienced psychological hypersensitivity regarding this cessation. I wondered if I was any less of woman without my cycle since the mere act of beginning menses represented a coming of age that shouted, "I AM NOW A WOMAN!" The loss of a menstrual cycle would, reasonably, mean that I was now LESS of a woman. Or, perhaps, was I woman at all? It's just blood. I wondered why blood between my legs would make me feel more or less like a woman. It then occurred to me that my menstruation was a metaphor for power and womanhood: blood inside the ring and blood between my legs.

When I began training less excessively and focused on my nutrition, my menstrual cycle began again. It was as if I had gotten it for the first time as a 13-year old, gasping in disbelief that I was healthy, growing, and womanly. My menstruation became a power tool-a secret weapon—that I believe resulted from the societal urgency to silence women's menstruation and women in general. Though I am no longer a competitive boxer, fitness and wellness have become my career and life's passion. My menstrual cycle has never been in jeopardy or posed a problem since I became healthy. However, my relationship with my cycle has shifted most prominently as it relates to the political and social climate of today.

As a result of the Presidential Election, the Women's March on Washington, and the #MeToo campaign, women have reclaimed a loud, proud, and powerful stance in the world. While men have been prosecuted for sexual misconduct toward women, women have taken to the streets to demand their political and social agency, rebuke anyone who fails to adhere to consent, and fight for equal rights (yes, something we still need to march for). Women are taking up space in the political stratosphere, much like a boxer will command inside the ring to shift power dynamics. The mere term "female boxer" depicts a dichotomy of competing gender norms: women engaging in bloody, barbaric sport. This same juxtaposition can be drawn for the women's movement. Using uncensored language, women have demanded power. My personal response to this movement has manifested itself in my relationship with my menstrual cycle. The inherent ability to menstruate might be reserved for females only, but the power associated with drawing blood has been likened to male aggression and power since the beginning of time. By reclaiming menstruation as a form of power and pride–menstrual anarchy as it were-we are redefining what it means to be women. Powerful women.

Seeing Red, White and Blue: The Patriotic Period

"War is menstrual envy."
(graffiti found in a women's bathroom stall)

Though simplistic, the epigraph above serves a purpose. It acts as a rebuke to the Freudian notion that women's discontent with their appointed roles can be summarized and dismissed as merely an expression of their lacking the male organ of potency: penis envy. The feminist psychoanalyst Karen Horney (1967) once claimed that the theory resulted from the fact that men need to disparage women more than women need to disparage men. She reversed the "penis envy" construct with the concept of "womb envy," another version of the idea that anatomical differences in genitalia held the keys to understanding human motivation, creativity, and fundamental psychology.

The graffiti takes the notion to another level, suggesting that rather than men envying the ability to give birth, to create life, they envy women's ability to bleed and not die. After all, all other mammals can give birth, but the human is a rarity in its ability to shed blood with little ill effect.

But the idea that at some deep, existential level male behavior in its most extreme form—banding together with one another in massive efforts to kill other bands of men in the savagery and ritual of war—is a crude attempt to emulate the monthly behavior of women, shedding blood and surviving its loss is, however whimsical or fantastical, an intriguing proposition. To the "pre-scientific" male observer, what could be more astounding, more desirable, than the ability to bleed and not die. And, after all, that is exactly what every individual who has ever gone into battle hopes for, to "come home alive" despite having lost some blood along the way and, thereby, earning heroic stature. Even those men (and they are virtually all men) who choose to martyr themselves in suicide bombings or other gestures of self-sacrifice do so in the belief that another life awaits them, that they will be "reborn" in a spiritual reenactment that emulates the workings of the menstrual cycle.

Having laid out this admittedly fanciful or even, to many readers, an extreme speculation of the formative influences of menstruation on one of the most universal of male institutions, war making, let us turn to specific examples of interfaces between menstruation and military endeavors.

A basic premise that underlies all of my work in the field of menstrual studies is that in patriarchal societies men have the power and authority to define the meaning of virtually every phenomenon, even biological and physical aspects of life that they themselves do not actually experience. Men were the creators of every

major world religion, of notions of the origins of life, of the body of art and literature that came to be called the canonical works. They even presumed to undertake
defining the meaning of being a woman, including the meaning of menstruation.
Menstrual bleeding has historically been a puzzling—even a miraculous—phenomenon in men's eyes. And though social and scientific progress has necessitated
significant adjustments in practice and belief, dealing with menstruation continues
to be a contested realm.

Since the turn of the millennium, American society has continued to redefine
the way it views women's bodies and minds relative to their fitness to perform tasks
that they have been historically and traditionally restricted from participating in,
including the opening of a wide range of military service options that had been
closed to women. In the past women were relegated to auxiliary realms of service,
especially military nursing, clerical work, and related fields. The full-scale mobi-
lization during World War II even led to a new set of designations and accompa-
nying acronyms. The Army had its WACS (Women in the Army Corp), the Navy
made WAVES (Women Accepted for Volunteer Emergency Service—a unit of
the Naval Reserve), and the Air Force had WAFs (Women in the Air Force). It
was deemed appropriate to identify these enlistees by their gender since it was
presumed that otherwise every "soldier" or "sailor" was a man. It was not necessary to use terms like MAC (Male in the Army Corp) or MEN (Male Enlisted
in the Navy) or MAF (Male in the Air Force). And since women were restricted
to service locations behind the lines of battle, the matter of access to menstrual
management did not arise.

Although the changes that have occurred in the 21st century reflect the success
of sociopolitical efforts to afford women greater equality and opportunity across
the full spectrum of social and economic engagement, they also are the result of
practical—one might even say cynical—decisions resulting from the elimination
of the military draft system and the need to fill the ranks of the armed services
with willing and qualified volunteers.

One of the most significant developments occurred in 2013 when Secretary
of Defense Leon Panetta, with the approval of the Joint Chiefs of Staff, lifted
all restrictions against women serving in combat positions. In fact, this ruling
merely recognized the reality that had already taken shape in the services as the
New York Times Magazine noted on March 18, 2007 with a cover story docu-
menting women's participation in combat situations and which later coverage
amply illustrated.

Debate over women's role in military service is complicated and cannot be
disposed of lightly. Given the history of gender stereotyping (of both men and
women) and role expectations, one can readily understand why placing men and

women in close quarters under treat of injury or death would require adjustments on everyone's part, not just those in the barracks and on the front lines. And since the menstrual cycle manifests itself in such vivid ways, it can easily become the synecdoche for larger questions as to how gender is constructed. An example of how this thinking works is noted by Zeigler and Gunderson (2005) who cite a male Army Major speaking at a conference as having "expressed concern, derisively, that bullets and MREs [meals-ready-to-eat] might be left behind so the 'ladies' could have Kotex" (p. 53).

The year following Panetta's decision that women could serve in combat, the Pentagon conducted a survey that concluded that most members of the armed forces had deeply held reservations about having women in their units and especially on the front lines. And while many of the doubts had to do with the distraction of female presence or whether women could to the job as well as men, as reported by Vagianos (2015), some of the comments in the survey specifically identified menstruation and PMS as the reason that women should not be in combat:

- "Acting on emotions may be a problem. Judgment may be altered. The effects of combat may have a different impact during those times, I'm not sure."—E-8, Air Force Special Operations Command
- "What about PMS and that time of the month? Do we just stock Midol and carry that around with us? There's nothing good about that."—E-8, Special Forces
- "I think PMS is terrible, possibly the worst. I cannot stand my wife for about a week out of the month for every month. I like that I can come to work and not have to deal with that."—E-6, Special Warfare Combatant Craft Crewman
- "I have a wife. She's very independent. But when that time of her month comes, she's weaker."—E-5, Navy SEAL (Vagianos, 2015).

The results of the Pentagon study also provoked reaction via a short, mocking video that was distributed via You Tube and other venues. Titled *Soldiers Period* and produced by Stotter and Rock (2016), the film features a number of women who had years of military experience. It consists of biting remarks by the women about how they had served in difficult circumstances and that their menstrual cycles had never diminished the quality of their performance.

Another demonstration of the changes that were taking place but also of how they were being depicted occurred in a Hollywood film directed by Ridley Scott and starring Demi Moore in 1997, *G.I. Jane.* The film captured male anxiety about having women in the ranks through a male soldier's anxious outburst,

"What about tampons?" and a reference to her developing amenorrhea due to the strenuous training regimen. However, I suspect that this detail might have been merely a plot device to avoid having to deal with menstrual management issues.

More recently, 2017 saw the publication of a memoir by Mary Jennings Hegar, *Shoot Like a Girl: One Woman's Dramatic Fight in Afghanistan and on the Home Front*. The book traces her combat experience as an Air Force pilot as well as her role as a plaintiff in the case that led to the elimination of the Ground Combat Exclusion Policy, the rule that was intended to keep women out of combat situations. As Hegar puts it, restrictions were meant to address "doomsday predictions of overly emotional women ruining the Air Force with their periods, babies, and breast milk..." (p. 280). Her book chronicles some of the menstrual barriers she faced such as the officer who belittled her because he believed that her menses might cause her to place others in peril, the cruel gynecological exam she was subject to, and encounters with other misogynist officers. (Building upon her military record and the exposure gained from the book's publication, Hegar went on to run for Congress in her home district in Texas.).

Underlying the effects of social changes such as the elimination of military conscription and the feminist movements' steady push for gender equality there are two related technical/medical developments: the birth control pill and menstrual suppression drugs. Pharmaceutical interventions in the menstrual cycle have had an immense impact on family planning, athletics, educational achievement, and employment, to name a few of the areas affected. In the realm of military service women can readily see how controlling or curtailing their ovulation can make it easier to perform their duties without having to cope with negative male attitudes and practical inconveniences. Menstrual suppression may also be seen as an aid to career advancement. Since the Department of Defense had set a 2016 goal of opening approximately 237,000 more positions to women, menstrual management has taken on a higher profile.

Arguments of how to best deal with the unique nature of the menstrual cycle within an institution that is so deeply steeped in male presumptions of physical needs and appropriate behavior as the military will not be easily resolved. In fact, the issues take on yet another layer of difficulty when women rise to positions of leadership and have to deal with officers from other countries' military establishments that have not made any accommodations to women's presence and that operate within very different systems of gender expectations. This is a topic that warrants, and will receive, continuing attention in the future.

Notes

1. A version of this review was originally published on the blog site *Menstruation Matters* on May 21, 2014, co-authored with Saniya Lee Ghanoui.
2. A version of this section was written by an amateur boxer, Robin Percyz, and originally appeared on the bog site of the Society for Menstrual Cycle Research, *Menstruation Matters*, on December 2, 2011.

References

Anon. (2009). Gibson blames "male menopause" for career slowdown. *Irish Examiner.* Retrieved July 3, 2017 from https://www.irishexaminer.com/breakingnews/entertainment/gibson-blames-male-menopause-for-career-slowdown-432028.html

Diamond, J. (1998). *Male menopause.* New York, NY: Penguin Random House.

Diamond, J. (2000). *Surviving male menopause: A guide for women and men.* New York, NY: Penguin Random House.

Diamond, J. (2010). *Mr. Mean: Saving your relationship from the irritable male syndrome.* San Rafael, CA: Vox Novus.

Freeman, D. (2010). Gibson blames temper on male menopause: Is he out of his mind? *CBSnews.* Retrieved on July 3, 2017 from https://www.cbsnews.com/news/mel-gibson-blames-temper-on-male-menopause-is-he-out-of-his-mind/

Fulbright, Y. (2009, September 09). FOXSexpert: Not such a myth: Male Menopause. *FoxNews.* Retrieved on July 3, 2017 from http://www.foxnews.com/story/2009/09/14/foxsexpert-not-such-myth-male-menopause.html

Gardner, T. (2013). "'Why are you harassing me?' Mel Gibson's rant at LA police as he is caught driving without his license on him." *MailOnline.* Retrieved on July 3, 2017 from https://www.google.com/search?q=Mel+Gibson's+road+rage&ie=utf-8&oe=utf-8&client=firefox-b-1-ab

Horney, K. (1967). *Feminine psychology.* New York, NY: W.W. Norton.

Marks, R. (Producer) & Jaglom, H. (Director). (2014). *The M Word* [Motion Picture]. United States: Breaking Glass Pictures.

Rock, M., & Stotter, E. (Producers & Directors). (2016). *Soldiers Period* [Video Production]. Retrieved on November 1, 2018 from http://www.menstruationresearch.org/2016/09/08/military-menses-you-dont-wanna-mess-with-this/

Scott, R. (Producer & Director). (1997). *G.I. Jane* [Motion Picture]. United States: Hollywood Pictures.

Vagianos, A. (2015). Elite combat troops deeply troubled by PMS. *Huffpost.* Retrieved on June 18, 2018 from https://www.huffingtonpost.com/entry/us-special-forces-completely-terrified-of-periods-women-in-general_us_56702043e4b0e292150f270b

Zeigler, S., & Gunderson, G. G. (2005). *Moving beyond G. I. Jane.* New York, NY: University Press of America.

Conclusion

Men in the Emerging Menstrual Ecology

The premise of this book has been that menstruation, while a biological characteristic of the human female's reproduction system, is also a socially and culturally constructed artifact of human invention. And though the physical act of menstruating, widely known as "having a period," is exclusive to those individuals with ovaries, hormone-producing glands, and other biological apparati, everyone, men and women alike, participates in crafting its meaning. It is with this premise in mind that I employ "menstrual transactions" as the term to describe the process through which individuals learn about, internalize, share, perpetuate, and challenge the definitions that constitute menstrual meaning. The previous chapters of this book have set out to examine the presence and workings of such transactions in settings ranging from ancient times to the recent past, as well as, and in some news media, literature, film, television, and advertising.

Every organic system, be it the evolution of species, technological developments, religions, political philosophies, and every other complex biological, sociological, or economic structure is made up of and responsive to a myriad of shifting influences. Such is also the case with the cultural, social and even the biological aspects of the menstrual cycle. Just as changes in diet, use of contraceptive technologies and other biological factors have altered the way the cycle functions, so have changes in the social arrangements of society altered attitudes and practices. I use the term "menstrual ecology" to refer to these dynamics in order to point out that menstruation exists within a constellation of ever-changing forces that shape and reshape the phenomenon's meaning in unpredictable ways. Though the term "ecology" is most commonly used in discussions of phenomena such as climate or the natural environment, its implication of interactivity makes it apt for discussion of the menstrual cycle as well.

The best example of the complexity of the menstrual ecology is found in the creation and wide adoption of the contraceptive device known as The Pill. No one anticipated the profound effect that this intervention in the workings of the female reproductive system would have on women's sense of their own sexuality as a result of their ability to take control of reproduction decisions. Even religious authority came into question as traditional faiths struggled with how to redefine the meaning of "contraception," a term that once meant interfering with a sperm's engagement with an egg during the act of intercourse. But was suspending ovulation itself really "contraception?" The ramifications of this nuance are still being felt.

Just as The Pill gave women, particularly young and unmarried women, the ability to control their menstrual cycles and thereby gave them greater control of their sex lives, and, therefore, the way men experienced sexual activity as well, at the other end of the age spectrum, another chemical/biological development has occurred more recently. The cessation of menstruation, menopause, has its own impact on women's sexual identity and activity. On one hand, as demonstrated in an episode of the television series *All in the Family*, discussed previously, some women feel a loss of sexual identity, especially if their sense of their own sexuality is rooted in the ability to conceive. For other women, the cessation of ovulation is liberating, as they no longer have to concern themselves with contraception and the relationship issues that pregnancy prevention entails. A negative effect, however, is that menopause is sometimes accompanied by a reduction in vaginal lubrication that can make sexual activity painful. This condition has led to the rise of various hormone replacement drugs that simulate the effects triggered by the glandular activity responsible for ovulation and related physical responses. One of the results is that women are able to experience pleasurable sexual relations more readily which, as an unanticipated consequence, suggests that men should be sexually active at later ages as well. The parallel developments of estrogen replacement products and erectile dysfunction drugs suggest the possibility that a subtle link exists between the two age-related factors that deserves further attention.

It has become axiomatic when examining the introduction of new technologies that there will be unanticipated consequences and this has certainly been the case with every effort to introduce new ways of managing the menstrual cycle. And the same holds true for changes in the political or economic climate. Consider the unintended effects of Donald Trump's election to the office of U.S. president upon the social menstrual ecology. As mentioned previously, Trump put menstruation on the political agenda when he implied that he was receiving unfair treatment from a woman journalist because (he presumed) she was probably menstruating. This comment (along with his recorded boast that he could get away with grabbing women's genitals) generated angry responses that included broadening the scope of acceptable discussions of women's reproductive processes and biology, including the menstrual cycle. In this case an unintended and unanticipated consequence was greater menstrual frankness.

Donald Trump's election (or, we might say Hillary Clinton's defeat) also led to the widely noted increase of women running for political office, not just for the highly visible Congressional positions and high-profile governor's slots but in races for state legislative positions and local offices. The election of women, and even the campaigns of those who lost, reshaped the political landscape. Greater women's presence in politics opens the door for the enactment of laws that pertain to the menstrual cycle. And it does not require that women be in the majority, only that women's interest be seen as of sufficient import that men in politics must vote on legislative proposals and be held accountable for their decisions.

There are two legislative initiatives that have become increasingly pressing. They are captured in a slogan that activists have used to dramatize the effort: "De-Tax & De-Tox the Tampon." The first part of the slogan refers to the drive to remove sales taxes from all menstrual products. In the U.S. this is a daunting task given the fragmented nature of sales tax levies. Unlike the practice in many other countries where tax policy is determined at the national level, every state and many local municipalities in America may decide what gets taxed and what does not. For instance, in Texas, menstrual products are taxed and Stetson cowboy hats are not. Pennsylvania may tax tampons but New Jersey might not. As a result, the political momentum behind the anti-tax drive is easily fragmented and localized.

The second part of the slogan refers to a bill that has been repeatedly introduced into the U.S. Congress by Congresswoman Carolyn Maloney known as The Robin Danielson Act. Named after a woman who died from toxic shock syndrome (TSS) due to the bleaching agents used in Rely tampons, the bill calls for stricter regulation and transparency in the manufacture of menstrual products so as to insure their safety. The act has languished in committee for more than a decade, but the election of more women would inevitably force it to a floor debate in Congress where male members would have to take public positions between increased government oversight of corporations and women's menstrual well-being.

Ironically, these initiatives following Donald Trump's election, are generated, in part, by response to the perception of an underlying misogyny. After all, the debate over abortion is basically a menstrual management issue, the matter of a missed period and how to respond to its absence. Pro-choice advocates want women to have the right to decide how to deal with the fact that they have stopped menstruating while anti-choice advocates contend that once a period has been missed due to the fertilization of an egg that women must relinquish the right to act in such a way as to place their bodies back into a regular menstrual cycle. Related questions were at the core of much of the controversy surrounding the nomination of Brett Kavanaugh to serve on the U.S. Supreme Court. When Senator Kamala Harris, asked the nominee, "Can you think of any laws that give the government the power to make decisions about the male body?" There was a long pause, some false starts, and a brief reply, "I'm not thinking of any right now, Senator" (Feller). In effect, Senator Harris had, without using a specific reference to the period, framed it as a matter of menstrual liberation and equity.

Beyond the realm of elections and legislation, political menstrual activism takes on other forms, one of which concerns pollution and environmental degradation. It seems unlikely that any single menstrual management device could have the far-reaching effects that the contraceptive pill has had on both women and men. Yet new devices come along and their full effect will be unknown for some time. Aside from variations on ovulation control systems such as drugs that fully suppress any sign of menstrual bleeding or intrauterine devices that prevent implantation or "morning after" pills that induce the shedding of uterine lining in case implantation has occurred, there are new methods of managing the presence of menstrual blood for those women who continue to have a menstrual cycle accompanied by monthly bleeding.

In this regard the steadily increasing interest in methods that have less impact on the natural environment is noteworthy. Environmental activists have found common cause with menstrual activists in confronting the negative effects of disposing thousands of plastic tampon applicators as well as used pads into landfills and ocean dumps. A side effect of these efforts has been that there is a greater awareness on the part of everyone concerned, regardless of gender, of the need to understand the workings of the menstrual cycle and how to attend to the disposal of the products used in its management.

Among the outcomes of increased awareness has been a new interest in the use of tampons that do not require applicators, reusable cloth pads, and especially menstrual cups, devices inserted into the uterus that collect menstrual fluid in a funnel-shaped silicone cup that is emptied and reused. Use of any of these products requires a greater familiarity and comfort with one's own body. It remains to be seen what the long-range effect of the new products will be both in terms of environment impact as well as interpersonal relations due to changes in menstrual attitudes.

As another way to get a sense of the unfolding trends, consider some menstrual news coverage over just a 10-month span in *The New York Times*. (The following examples constitute a random sample and are less than comprehensive.):

October 21, 2017—a lengthy profile of Chirlane McCray, New York City Mayor Bill De Blasio's wife, began on the front page and continued for a full page inside. Among the noteworthy details that the (male) writer thought would capture McCray's activist, outspoken personality was mention of an item on her blog about the importance of providing menstrual products in schools and a poem she wrote on the topic. (Goldmacher, p. A-1)

November 5, 2017—In a profile of the actor/producer Laurence Fishburne the interviewer, Kathryn Shattuck, began a question about his new show by stating, "On *black-ish* the show has dealt with police brutality, the presidential election and even menstruation." Though Fishbourne did not comment on the presence of a menstrual element in the show, the fact that the reporter thought it worth mentioning is a departure from the kind of topics that would have been included just a few years previously, especially in an interview of a male celebrity by a female reporter. (Shattuck, p. D-2)

January 11, 2018—An article was previewed on page one by a color photograph with the caption, "Many women in rural Nepal sleep outdoors during menstruation, putting lives at risk." Inside, on page 4, the full piece, co-authored by a man, was titled, "In Nepal, a Taboo Claims Another Victim." It reported on "...a very old tradition in rural Nepal in which religious Hindus believe that menstruating women are unclean and should be banished from the family home." Due to the severity of the weather and the danger of poisonous snakes that sometimes are found in menstrual huts, the article states that, "...dozens of women and girls have died in recent years from following this tradition, despite activists' campaigns and government efforts to end the practice." There is a subtle tone in the report that carries a sense of condescension toward the backward people in rural Nepal who cannot bear the presence of a menstruating woman while American readers (at least *New York Times* readers, men and women alike) are completely at ease. The contrast is dramatized by the inclusion of a large photograph of a tiny hut with two women and their young daughters huddled under blankets. (Sharman, p. A-4)

April 1, 2018—An essay in the "Sunday Review" section of the *Times*, written by former Society for Menstrual Cycle Research President, Chris Bobel, was titled "When Pads Can't Fix Prejudice." This piece discussed the importance of thinking beyond the notion that simply providing menstrual products to girls and women would adequately address the taboos and superstitions surrounding the period. Bobel calls for a more comprehensive approach: "Challenging the social stigma and disgust directed at the female body must be our main mission—in the developing world and everywhere else." The significance of the essay is not just its content but that it is found in the august pages of the op-ed section of the *New York Times*, one of the most widely read and influential publications in America that is assumed to be consumed by men as well as women. (Bobel, p. SR-9)

August 30, 2018—In the "International" portion of the *Times*, at the top of page 5, an item titled "Scotland Plans to Offer Free Sanitary Products to Students" reported that, "Scotland has become the first country to provide free sanitary products to students at schools, colleges and universities, an effort to banish 'period poverty,' in which girls and women miss out on their studies because they cannot afford protection." The article goes on to discuss the fact that other countries are considering similar actions including the removal of the 5% sales tax on sanitary products; however, there is a policy within the European Union that classifies such products as "luxury, nonessential" items that may not be exempt. A good example of unanticipated consequences also appeared: an effort to funnel the millions raised in taxes on menstrual products into women's charities was met with outrage because it implied that only women were being taxed to provide the benefit. (Yeginsu, p. 5+)

August 31, 2018—The day after the report on menstrual developments in Scotland, the *Times* reported on a case of menstrual mischief in France under the headline, "Protesting Paris Urinals as Sexist, Vandals Use Tampons, Graffiti and Cement." Efforts to address the problem of men urinating on the streets of Paris had led to the installation of items known as "eco-toilets," waist high boxes with openings through which men could relieve themselves in public places, including along the Seine beside a public pathway. The fact that there were no similar accommodations for women to use led to acts of urinal vandalism including plastering the objects with tampons. The article did not mention if the tampons were used ones. (Breeden, p. A-7)

September 2, 5 & 6, 2018—Within a five day span the *Times* ran three prominently placed photos of women dressed in the red robes and white cowls that are the costumes of the fertile women in Margaret Atwood's *Handmaid's Tale*. The first was to illustrate an op-ed piece (Paltrow, p. SR-7) in the Sunday Review section about the possible effects of repeal of Roe v. Wade; the next was on the front page (above the fold!) to accompany coverage of the Senate appearance of Judge Brett Kavanaugh (Stolberg & Liptak, p. A-1); the third was a shot of women in Handmaid garb protesting a legislative initiative in Texas that would require the cremation of any fetal tissue produced during an abortion (Fernandez, p. A-16). The image of groups of women wearing the costumes of the characters in the successful series based on Atwood's novel has become one of the dominant metaphors for those attacking misogynist policies. The novel reduces gender politics to a matter of menstrual management and use of its imagery as an activist symbol is intended to point out the contradiction between valuing women for their reproductive capacity while at the same time reducing them to menstrual machines whose purpose is a mechanical one.

Beyond the pages of *The New York Times* other media have also expanded the presence of menstrual references as in the following examples:

- An item carried by the Associated Press and reported in the September 23, 2017 issue of *The Charlotte Observer* reported, "Miss Turkey dethroned over 'unacceptable' tweet." The pageant winner, Itir Essen, was stripped of her title because she tweeted a political statement referring to the previous year's coup attempt. She wrote, "I got my period on the morning of July 15 martyrs' day. I'm marking the day by bleeding as a representation of the martyr's blood" (Anon, p. 2A). It was not clear if the punishment was only due to the menstrual detail or because of its implicit support of the failed coup.
- Even the cartoon pages have opened the menstrual closet. The cartoon, "Between the Lines" drawn by Max Garcia for the *New York Daily News* depicted a menstrual pad with wings flying through the sky while shouting "Up, up and awaaaay!" On the ground below a little tampon says, "Boy, I wish I could fly." This may not be the funniest gag imaginable, but the fact that a pad and tampon joke appeared in the cartoon pages of a widely circulated daily paper suggests that the menstrual ecology is undergoing change. (Garcia, p. 32)
- Lest one think that the American Association of Retired People (AARP) is focused solely on advocating for Social Security and various geriatric causes, the August/September, 2018 issue devoted more that six pages to menstrual concerns in a feature titled, "What Doctors Don't Know About Menopause" (Wolff, p. 37+). This is yet another indication that the once taboo topic is now considered worthy of inclusion in a publication that is distributed to both women and men with no need for coy evasions of its content.

On still another front, consider the world of poetry. Contrast the pristine universe of Robert Frost's "The Road Not Taken," for example, with Sharon Olds' collection published in 2016, simply titled *Odes*. Along with titles such as "Ode to the Hymen," "Ode to the Condom," and "Blow Job Ode," one finds "Ode to the Tampon," "Ode to Menstrual Blood" and "Ode for the Vagina" (Olds, 2016). It is not just that a woman would be bold enough to write such titles, but that Sharon Olds is a widely regarded poet, winner of the most prestigious literary recognition, including the Pulitzer Prize for poetry, the T.S. Eliot Prize and the National Book Critics Circle Award, to name just a few. The participation of men in making such decisions means that her work is widely read and its content becomes a factor in shaping both women's and men's understanding (and in this case, their appreciation) of the nuances of the menstrual cycle. Poetry at its best is a literary genre that provokes, confronts, and challenges. Sharon Olds in this regard is a menstrual provocateur. When it comes to using tampons, for instance, many men are completely clueless. But with her tampon ode and other genital-themed poems Olds gives men a glimpse into the foreign world of the vagina that they would otherwise be unlikely to have. And although these works are probably not being taught at the high school level, their inclusion in college literature classes is sure to have effects, though they cannot easily be measured.

As all of these examples illustrate, menstrual news is no longer consigned to the menstrual closet, the ghetto of the "women's pages" or to targeted magazines like *Cosmopolitan*. Increasingly, menstrual news items are thought to be of "general" interest, that is, of interest to men too.

Another avenue for entry into the menstrual ecology is via the menstrual economy, a fact that the editors at *Forbes* have recognized. On February 9, 2018, they published on line an item titled, "Why Bollywood's 'Pad Man' Is Getting India Talking About Periods" (Mangaldas). It described a new film about a man named Arunachalam Muruganantham who has garnered a great deal of attention for championing women's access to inexpensive, disposable menstrual pads. He has become the darling of some menstrual activist circles as the "sensitive male" who, in sympathy for his wife being forced to use dirty rags to manage her period because they could not afford commercial sanitary napkins, invented a machine to create low cost pads from local plant material. The coverage of his story has repeatedly focused on the economic aspects of the story. He has become a New Age Midas, a man who can turn blood into gold.

A few months later (August 31, 2018) *Forbes* returned to the subject with "How One Woman Is Starting A Menstrual Revolution In Kenya" (Bloom), an extended interview with Megan White Mukuria, the founder of ZanaAfrica, an organization based in Kenya dedicated to providing menstrual health education as well as locally produced, inexpensive menstrual products. In keeping with the *Forbes* focus on business, the article begins by pointing out that, "In 2016, the feminine hygiene product market was worth $23 billion…. And it is expected to grow to $32 billion in 2022." Placing a discussion of the role of menstruation in the context of educational and employment opportunities for girls and women shifts it away from that of intimate details of the female reproductive system thereby making it of suitable interest for male readers. Businessmen interested in investment opportunities and entrepreneurial possibilities would have to develop greater knowledge of just how the menstrual cycle works, how many pads a woman might purchase over her life time, the pros and cons of tampon use in the context of religious and social restrictions, how to advertise products within a given social setting, and how to make one's own brand more appealing. All of these factors require men to engage with women more openly in order to gain a higher level of understanding of aspects of the period that might impact manufacturing, distribution, and sales.

The effect of these developments—and many more not mentioned—has been to move menstruation from the margins into the mainstream. The outcome is to place new challenges and opportunities before men. Some will resist pressures for greater awareness and acceptance of a "fact of life" they have managed to avoid or to control; others will embrace the invitation to engage actively in the shaping of the rules, regulations and rituals of the menstrual ecology; most will "go with the flow," as it were, integrating new perspectives into their relationships and value systems as required or convenient.

There is nothing static about the menstrual ecology, and menstrual transactions will continue to be sources of fascination in ways both large and small. Consider one final example. *The New York Times* is sometimes referred to as "The Grey Lady" for its role as "the newspaper of record" and its reportorial rectitude. The Sunday *Times* magazine has for seven decades included a large crossword puzzle that has a dedicated following of puzzlers. As a long-time puzzle solver myself, to the best of my knowledge, menstruation has been an off limits topic for clues and answers. But on October 27, 2018, that line was crossed when frequent puzzle designer Erik Agard included a clue that might have been a stumper years ago but in recent times probably found many quick solutions, especially among the women working the puzzle grid. The clue was for a six letter word answer to 62 Down: "Pad alternative." The speed with which one could fill in the squares was a sign of one's menstrual awareness as well as one's puzzle skills (Agard, p. 72).

References

Agard, E. (2018, October 27). Match play. *The New York Times Sunday Magazine*. p. 72.

Anon. (2017, September 23). Miss Turkey dethroned over "unacceptable" tweet. *The Charlotte Observer*, p. A2.

Bloom, L. (2018, August 31). How one woman is starting a menstrual revolution in Kenya. *Forbes*. Retrieved September 6, 2018, from https://www.forbes.com/sites/laurabegley bloom/2018/08/31/woman-starting-menstrual-revolution-kenya/#1db66b722044

Bobel, C. (2018, April 1). When pads can't fix prejudice. *The New York Times*, p. SR9.

Breeden, A. (2018, August 31). Protesting Paris urinals as sexist, vandals use tampons, graffiti and cement. *The New York Times*, p. A7.

Feller, M. (2018, September 6). Senator Kamala Harris stumped Brett Kavanaugh with a question about abortion. *Elle*. Retrieved September 6, 2018, from https://www.elle.com/culture/career-politics/a23006495/senator-kamala-harris-brett-kavanaugh-abortion-question-confirmation-hearings/

Fernandez, M. (2018, September 6). Federal judge rejects a Texas law requiring cremation of fetal tissue. *The New York Times*, p. A16.

Garcia, M. (2017, August 4). Between the lines (cartoon). *New York Daily News*, p. 32.

Goldmacher, S. (2017, October 21). In New York, an influential first lady with plans of her own. *The New York Times*, p. A1+.

Mangaldas, L. (2018, February 9). Why Bollywood's "PadMan" is getting India talking about periods. Retrieved September 6, 2018, from https://www.forbes.com/sites/leezaman galdas/2018/02/09/why-bollywoods-pad-man-is-getting-india-talking-about-peri ods/#ac56d894879f

Olds, S. (2016). *Odes*. New York, NY: Alfred A. Knopf.

Paltrow, L. (2018, September 2). Life after Roe. *The New York Times*, p. SR7.

Sharman, B., & Gettleman, J. (2018, January 11). In Nepal, a taboo claims another victim. *The New York Times*, p. A4.

Shattuck, K. (2017, November 5). Laurence Fishburne's role made him cry. *The New York Times*, p. D2.

Stolberg, S., & Liptak, A. (2018, September 5). Democrats hurl fierce barrage at court choice. *The New York Times*, p. A1.

Wolff, J. (2018, August/September). What doctors don't know about menopause. *AARP the Magazine*, p. 37+.

Yeginsu, C. (2018, August 30). Scotland plans to offer free sanitary products to students. *The New York Times*, p. A5.

Index

P

Panetta, Leon, 172
Parker-Bowles, Camilla,
   2, 55–60, 62
Parton, Dolly, 142–143
Patchett, Ann, 66–68, 70
The Patron Saint of Liars, 68
Personal Products Advertising Guidelines,
   129–131
The Pill, 150–154, 178
Pliny, 20
"PMS" (song), 28, 147
"PMS Blues," 141–144, 149
Pope Gregory, 50–51
pre-menstrual phase, 9, 18, 19, 143–144
Prince Charles, 2, 12, 15, 55–62
Princess Diana, 56, 61–62
Pulp Fiction, 116, 118

Q

Qaddafi, 18
Quran, 24

R

Rachel (biblical), 39–46, 158–159
The Rage: Carrie 2, 107
Reagan, Ronald, 19
The Red Tent, 43–45
Robbins, Tom, 65
Robin Danielson Act, 179
Roe v. Wade, 83, 182
Romeo and Juliet, 19, 55, 74–75, 113
Roseanne, 84, 85
Rosemary's Baby, 104–105
Roth, Philip, 70, 72–75
Run, 68

S

Sabbath's Theater, 72–74
Scotland, 182
Secrets and Lies, 119
Seeger, Pete, 151
self-pity, 146
7th Heaven, 86
Sex, Literature and Censorship, 62
Sex and the City, 83–84
sexual education, 4, 30, 32, 94, 115
Shakespeare, William, 9, 17–18, 19, 62, 75,
   113–114
Sherman Anti-Trust Act, 129
Shoot Like a Girl, 174
Sixteen Candles, 115–116
Smile, 106–109
soap operas, 128
social amenorrhea, 23
Soldier's Period, 173
Sophocles, 39, 43
Soul Stirrers, The, 148
Sorority Life, 158–159
Sotomayor, Sonia, 19
South Park, 82, 93–97, 99, 116, 156
Sparks, Donita, 25–26, 160
Spencer, Diana, 56
Spencer, Scott, 65, 70, 74–75, 113–114
Standards and Practices policies, 129
State of Wonder, 66, 67
Steinem, Gloria, 163
Superbad, 120
"Superman," 148
Supreme Court, 19, 83, 180
"Sympathy Pains," 135–137

T

taboos, 9, 11, 36, 43–44, 47, 50–51, 60, 71–72,
   74–76, 82–83, 87, 89, 91, 94, 105, 107, 111,
   113, 120, 156–161, 163, 169, 181, 183

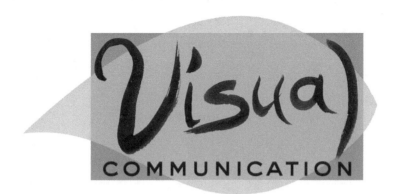

Susan B. Barnes, *General Editor*

Visual communication is the process through which individuals in relationships, organizations, and cultures interpret and create visual messages in response to their environment, one another, and social structures. This series seeks to enhance our understanding of visual communication, and explores the role of visual communication in culture. Topics of interest include visual perception and cognition; signs and symbols; typography and image; research on graphic design; and the use of visual imagery in education. On a cultural level, research on visual media analysis and critical methods that examine the larger cultural messages imbedded in visual images is welcome. By providing a variety of approaches to the analysis of visual media and messages, this book series is designed to explore issues relating to visual literacy, visual communication, visual rhetoric, visual culture, and any unique method for examining visual communication.

For additional information about this series or for the submission of manuscripts, please contact Dr. Barnes at *susanbbarnes@gmail.com.*

To order other books in this series, please contact our Customer Service Department:

(800) 770-LANG (within the U.S.)
(212) 647-7706 (outside the U.S.)
(212) 647-7707 FAX

Or browse online by series at www.peterlang.com.